IRIDOLOGY
in PRACTICE

Revealing the
Secrets of the Eye

Praise for Dr. Miriam Garber and

Iridology in Practice

"I have read *Iridology in Practice: Revealing the Secrets of the Eye*. [This] wonderful work and [the author's] broad knowledge have created a synthesis of the various aspects of eye diagnosis that will, without doubt, bring great blessing to the public thirsting for this knowledge. I have observed that the wealth of suggestions and [Garber's] interesting guidance are the foundations of this system and their influence is significant. I am sure that [this] book will contribute much to improving the general public's knowledge and practitioner's knowledge of complementary medicine and will promote relief and healing."

—Dr. Shlomo Shlezinger,
The Center of Human Behaviour

"Any new publication in the field of iridology is to be celebrated and particularly one with such a diverse approach, historical basis, and new challenging material. This book carries a wealth of experience and the content I have seen is excellent, practical, and pushes us out of the comfort zone we may find ourselves in from time to time. This is vital in the field of iridology and helps the professional progression continue on a global scale. It is an honour and privilege to be able to write these words . . . and I recommend this book for all involved in natural health and iridology. The emphasis here is true holistic health and is a most welcome addition to iridology literature."

—John Andrews, England • November 2007

"We are happy to have our Iris Diagnosis Chart published in this book. This chart was developed, edited, and printed in Hebrew, in Israel, by Dr. Mordechai Netzach [pioneer of natural practitioners and instructors of healthy living and self-healing in Israel] and has been distributed since 1942. Dr. Netzach helped many on the path to health with this noninvasive method and taught some of them to work professionally with this wonderful, accurate, and efficient method and to continue his work with coming generations. Iridology, which was a large part of his life's work in addition to other methods of natural therapy, was another step towards fulfilling his dream, that continues to come true, and the dream of others who share his vision, all over the world."

—Miriam Netzach, widow of Dr. Mordechai Netzach,
Shlomit Netzach, and family

IRIDOLOGY
in PRACTICE

*Revealing the
Secrets of the Eye*

Miriam Garber, Ph.D., MBMD, Dip.H.Ir.

Basic
Health
PUBLICATIONS, INC.

Photos by Dr. Miriam Garber. Pictures on pages 17–42 and instructional material on pages 18–42 used by permission of Professor Heinz W. Schmidt.

Translated from Hebrew to English by Judy Granit.

Iris Diagnosis Chart on page xv developed by Dr. Mordechai Netzach.

The thoughts and quotations in this book are provided courtesy of Avi Yacobovich, a natural nutrition counselor, author, and editor of *Aluma*—a weekly natural medicine magazine published in Israel.

A version of this book was printed in Tel-Aviv, Israel, by Contento de Semrikin in 2008. Proofreading and editing by Jonathan Danilowitz; Professional medical editing by Dr. Henia Lichter, M.D.; Graphic design by Studiomooza.

Basic Health Publications, Inc.
www.basichealthpub.com

Published by arrangement with Contento de Semrik, Tel-Aviv, Israel.

Library of Congress Cataloging-in-Publication Data

Garber, Miriam, author.
  Iridology in practice : revealing the secrets of the eye / Miriam Garber.
    p. ; cm.
  Includes bibliographical references and index.
  ISBN 978-1-59120-360-5 (Pbk.)
  ISBN 978-1-68162-741-0 (Hardcover)
  I. Title.
  [DNLM: 1. Eye Manifestations. 2. Iris—pathology. 3. Complementary Therapies—
  4. Diamethods.gnostic Techniques, Ophthalmological. 5. Sclera—pathology. WW 240]
  RE352
  617.7'2075—dc23
                                                    2013038410

Editor: Carol Killman Rosenberg
Typesetting/Layout: Gary A. Rosenberg
Cover design: Mike Stromberg

Contents

APPENDICES

"If I have seen further it is by standing on the shoulders of giants."

—SIR ISAAC NEWTON

With love to my mother, Leah;
may she rest in peace.

IRIS DIAGNOSIS CHART—מפת אבחון האירידס

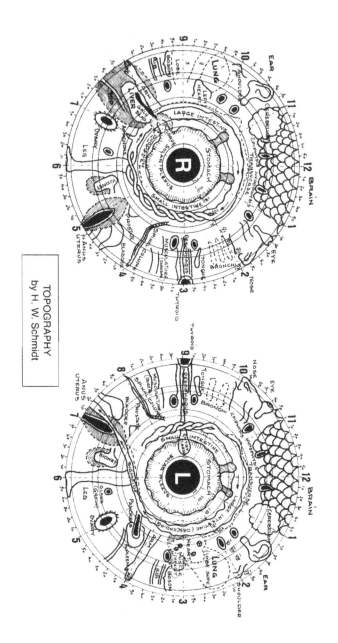

TOPOGRAPHY
by H. W. Schmidt

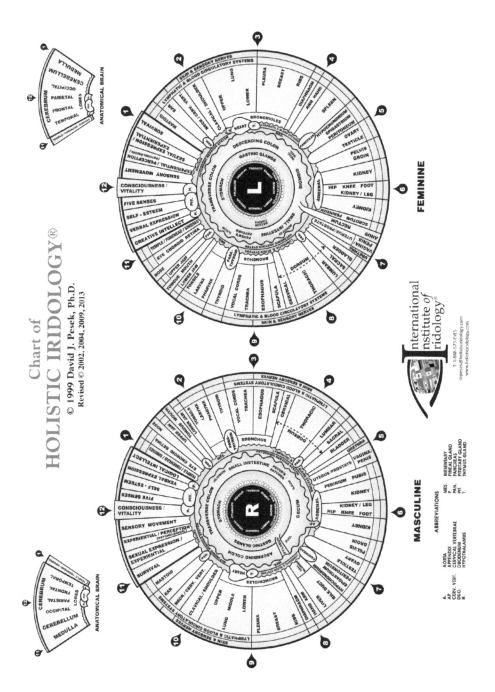

Chart of
HOLISTIC IRIDOLOGY®
© 1999 David J. Pesek, Ph.D.
Revised © 2002, 2004, 2009, 2013

IRIDOLOGY CHART

Developed by Bernard Jensen, D.C., Ph.D. with revisions by Ellen Jensen, Ph.D., D.Sc.

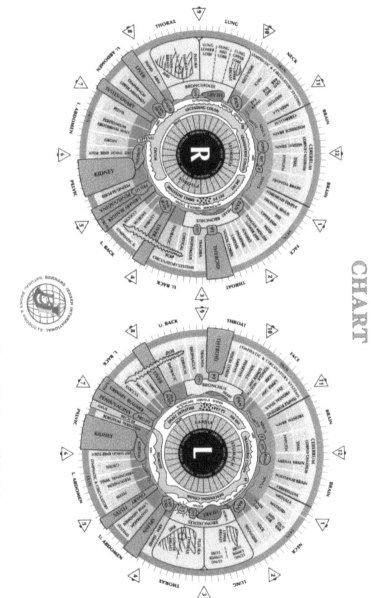

Acknowledgments

My deepest gratitude to Dr. Shlomo Shlezinger, who generously shared his boundless knowledge with me, helping me immeasurably in moments of doubt when dealing with my clients' complex problems. Thank you for putting your complete trust in me, helping me to grow and flourish, and for instilling in me my love of this profession.

To my friend Zahava Danziger, my heartfelt thanks to a special lady who shared my misgivings and decisions. Thank you for your pointed criticism, your razor-sharp thoughts, and your love and frankness that echoed inside me and were a guiding light over the years.

Thank to my close friend Nurit Shtreichman, for encouraging me to write, for revealing the secrets of the computer to me, and for giving of her time and energy to process the lovely photographs illustrating this book.

To Ora Zilberberg, my beloved friend, thank you for being a "lighthouse" shining bright light on foggy days along the paths of my life.

To Dr. Eric Pearl and the group of chosen scientists: Thanks to them, I acquired a new way of viewing life and the universe.

To my children, some of whom joined me on this voyage and who are my most exacting teachers.

To my grandchildren, whose love and smiles bring great light to my life.

Thanks, too, to all my clients, who put their trust in me and inspired me with their extraordinary ideas; to all my students—I have learned from you all; and, last but not least, to my husband, Hagai: thank you for your support and the encouragement that allowed me to devote myself to study and growth.

To the friends who are at my side.

To God who is with me.

Introduction

Iridology is a diagnostic method based on science and philosophy —*science* because the markings can be accurately interpreted, and *philosophy* because diagnosis is based on the observer's knowledge and personal analysis. The iridologist's ability to see in depth influences the interpretation of the markings. This system can be used to read a person's physical, emotional, and mental state by the color, tissue density, and markings on the iris (the colored part of the eye).

Iridology in Practice: Revealing the Secrets of the Eye focuses on teaching this system and offering qualified practitioners a useful and efficient tool. In this book, I pass on the valuable knowledge I gained from my teachers and have gathered through years of experience, observation, and research. I had the opportunity and privilege to practice my art and examine thousands of eyes and to understand and develop my own point of view.

Iridology is a powerful tool. As explained in this book, practitioners should know how to use the collected information for the client's maximum benefit. The professional iridologist's work stems from devotion and in-depth knowledge, combined with humility and respect for the client. I recommend that clients be treated lovingly and compliantly without judgment or prejudice. A client should be viewed as a person who is requesting assistance. Of course, the client must take responsibility for his or her own healing, even if we, the practitioners, have the means to help. Our job is to accompany clients on their path to health, to shed light on the dark spots in their lives, to be guides and teachers, and, if our assistance is desired, to be there for them all the way toward health.

The accuracy of this method enables us to delve into the deepest levels of the client's personality and to better understand his or her motives in choosing a lifestyle. For this reason, this knowledge should be used with the greatest of care. Beyond the technical aspects of iridology, this book presents a holistic approach to body, mind, and soul.

Please keep in mind that iridology is only a diagnostic tool. This book presents methods of treating and improving various states through methods I have learned and experienced in many fields of complementary medicine. You may use additional methods from your own "toolbox."

I wish success and fulfillment to everyone setting out on this fascinating journey.

PART ONE

Iridology Explained

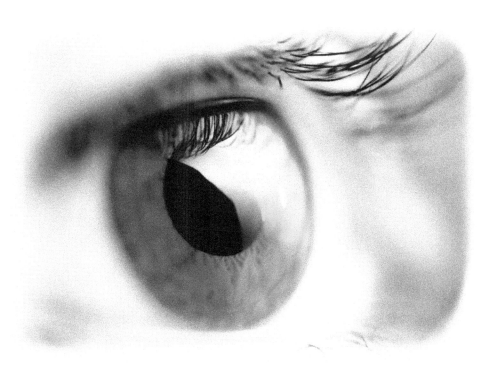

⬬ ⬬ ⬬ ⬬ ⬬ ⬬

CHAPTER 1

What Is Iridology?

Iridology is the science of observing and identifying markings in the iris (the colored part of the eye). These markings represent a person's genetic blueprint and congenital characteristics and offer a means of evaluating the functioning of various organs in the body. The following states can be detected through observation and identification: congenital weaknesses, inflammation, changes in the structure of tissues, susceptibility to diseases, the existence of disease-related conditions, the accumulation of toxins, and more. Above all, observing the iris offers insight into a person's lifestyle, including the damage caused by an unsuitable lifestyle for that person.

WHY MARKINGS APPEAR IN THE EYE AND HOW THEY CORRESPOND TO THE BODY

The physical body contains a large, complex web of nerves that originate in the organs, connect through the spine, and terminate in the brain. Information from every cell in the body flows through the nervous system to the brain and is permanently stored in the cellular memory. Computers store information on their data-storage disk and display the information on a monitor for us to see. Similarly, in the human body, the nervous system stores information and the eyes serve as a monitor, displaying markings that correspond to what is happening in the body.

The ability to identify the markings, link the information with the location of the various organs shown on the iridology chart, and the skill of combining knowledge of the body's pathology with this information enables us to use the data displayed in the eye to diagnose how the body is functioning. It may seem complicated, but in practice, it is quite simple. Iridology enables us to do a quick, painless, noninvasive data check, using simple tools.

While iridologists read the markings in the eye, the eye is not regarded as a visual organ in this system, and we do not treat visual disorders. Iridologists regard the eye as a "window" or "monitor" that reflects all the body's organs and systems, including the visual system. As such, eye disorders are displayed in the area corresponding to the eye on the iridology chart. The markings at that location indicate the severity of any damage.

Iridology can give us an exact picture of the cause of a client's ailments. In cases of chronic disease, iridology enables us to accurately estimate the degree of tissue damage and damage to a specific organ or to the entire system.

Iridology can be used to estimate a client's stress and anxiety levels. Furthermore, we can reveal the exact age at which traumas that left their mark in the psyche or physical body occurred. Other fascinating information we can glean from the eye is a client's emotional/psychological state and his or her everyday functioning at all levels of existence.

Contrary to Western medicine's "mechanical" approach in which the body is seen as a collection of organs to be treated separately by doctors specializing in each organ (for example, a cardiologist for coronary disorders, an orthopedist for the skeletal system, a gynecologist for women's reproductive health, and so on), iridologists regard a person as a whole—a totality of body/psyche/spirit that cannot be split into separate entities. If something happens on one level, it instantly affects the next level in descending order: psyche/mind to emotion and then to the physical body.

Another advantage of iridology analysis is the ability to discover a client's susceptibility to a certain disorder long before the disorder manifests itself, allowing for preventive medicine.

WHAT IRIDOLOGY CAN AND CANNOT REVEAL

What Iridology Can Reveal

- Constitution—potential of the congenital structure
- Organ and system weakness, including glandular functioning
- Genetics—the organism's inherited characteristics
- Hyperactivity and hypoactivity of organs/glands
- Biochemical processes
- Absorption level of vital substances
- Functioning level of the twelve bodily systems (see Appendix B)
- Blood circulation, blood quality
- Calcification of blood vessels plus cholesterol
- Diabetic tendency
- Deficiency of vitamins and minerals
- Toxicity levels of various bodily systems
- The effects of an organ on other organs
- Metabolism
- Inflammation
- Acidity/alkalinity
- Level of resistance to disease
- Parasites
- Precancerous indications
- Emotional states
- Traumatic periods and their influence on organs

What Iridology Cannot Reveal

- If a disease is present in the body

- Eye disorders

- Blood pressure levels, high or low (can be read in the sclera)

- Presence of a tumor (can be read in the sclera)

- Blood cholesterol levels

- Blood sugar level

- Type of parasite (can been read in the sclera)

- Level of candida activity

- Gender

- Pregnancy

THE HISTORY OF IRIDOLOGY

The study of eye markings originated in Asia thousands of years ago. More intensive research occurred during the sixteenth century. While German researchers, including Johann Eltzholtz and Philippus Meyens, published papers on eye markings prior to the nineteenth century, the first serious breakthrough was made by Ignatz von Peczely, a Hungarian doctor (1826–1911).

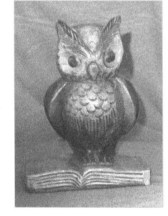

At the age of eleven, von Peczely freed a trapped owl in his garden. The owl's leg had been fractured, and he noticed a black line in the lower part of the owl's iris. He tended the owl's leg, and after three weeks, he noticed that a white line now appeared where the black line had been. Von Peczely concluded that there was a connection between what had happened to the owl's leg and the marking in its eye, and this aroused his curiosity. As an adult, he studied medicine and qualified as a doctor at the age of forty-one.

Von Peczely opened a homeopathic clinic in Budapest and began to research the link between bodily occurrences and iris markings. This laid the foundation for modern iridology. The many patients von Peczely examined during his work in the hospital afforded him an excellent opportunity to cross-check information read in the eye with various illnesses. He recorded the markings in patients' irises before and after surgery and found a positive correlation between information read in the eye and physical pathology.

At the same time, doctors and researchers in various fields of natural medicine in different countries were researching the link between eye markings and bodily organs. Eventually, a topographic map of the eye was developed, recording the relative position of the various organs. A picture of the body's condition can be obtained by deciphering these markings and their positioning on the map of the iris.

The System Presented in this Book

This book presents a combination of the system of iridology developed by Professor Heinz W. Schmidt and that developed by Dr. Bernard Jensen.

Professor Schmidt, the former president of the European Association of Natural Healing Practitioners (UEHP) and president of the Association of International Schools of Traditional Medicine (ISTM), currently heads a school of natural medicine in Saarbrucken, Germany. Dr. Bernard Jensen, now deceased, founded a school and healing center, which is still in operation. His successor, Dr. Ellen Tart Jensen, is past president of the International Iridology Practitioners Association (IIPA)—an association of which I have been a member for several years. The Association holds annual conferences for iridologists from around the world, who share up-to-date information from various research projects to enhance the knowledge of all participants.

There is a fundamental difference between Dr. Jensen's and Professor Schmidt's systems:

Professor Schmidt focuses on the congenital structure (constitution) as established by eye color and additional identifying markings. His system enables us to glean maximum information on the subject's health status in minimum time. The information is focused and amazingly accurate. As soon as we establish the subject's constitution, we can tell which weaknesses accompany him or her through life. The constitution's components provide an explanation of the source of many symptoms described in clients' complaints. On the other hand, Dr. Jensen's system focuses on specific markings that reflect the functioning of the various bodily systems in great detail. The process of gleaning this information is far more time-consuming but worth the effort.

Over the years I have honed my skill in combining both systems in my work. This allows me to build a broad picture of the information contained in the iris. Combining these methods increases my ability to give a comprehensive answer to the various problems my clients present. Nevertheless, this book focuses largely on Professor Schmidt's method, which is based on knowledge from his predecessors, including Josef Deck, as well as on his own research and development. According to Professor Heinz W. Schmidt:

> Iridology gives us beyond all diagnostic methods a very comprehensive, constitutional diagnosis where we recognize any organic deficiency. This leads to preventive measures or treatments long before any acute dysfunction, e.g., long before any state of acute ailment.
>
> The constitutions are genotypes; therefore, they are hereditary protons that cannot be changed.
>
> But lifestyle can be changed—dietary habits, sleep, place of residence, stress level, relationships—so as to strengthen the body, minimize congenital weaknesses and prevent development. It is my opinion that Iridology deserves to be incorporated in the diagnostic procedures of medicine.

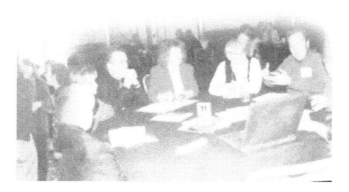

IIPA Conference USA, 2005

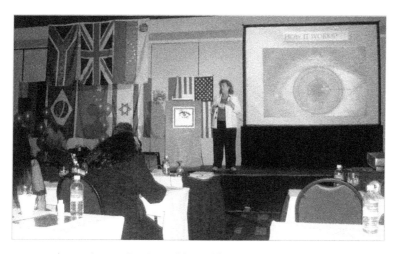

Lecturing at the 2011 Ohio, USA, Iridology Congress

ANATOMY OF THE EYE

The eyes are the visual organs of humans and animals. The eyeball rests in the eye socket and includes both the sclera and the iris. There are six socket muscles surrounding the eyeball. Their purpose is to move it. A tear system lubricates the frontal part of the eye.

The human eyeball is approximately 24 mm in diameter and has three main layers:

1. The outer, protective layer

2. The central, vascular layer

3. The inner, sensory layer

The cornea is composed of five layers. The outer layer is the epithelium. The cornea's transparency is achieved through all its components sharing the same refractive index.

The middle layer of the eyeball is composed of the choroid, the cilliary body, and the iris. The cilliary body is ring shaped and supports the lens and changes its shape. The choroid is composed of many blood vessels, pigment cells, and connective tissue. The iris is composed of connective tissue, blood vessels, and radial and peripheral muscles that control the size of the pupil. This tissue is called stroma.

The third and deepest layer is the retina.

Eye muscles – left eye

Superior oblique

Superior rectus

Optic nerve

Medial rectus

Lateral rectus

Inferior oblique

Inferior rectus

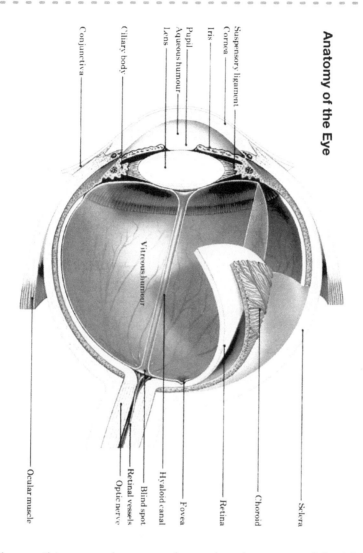

Chapter 13

Anatomy of the Eye

Conjunctiva
Ciliary body
Lens
Aqueous humour
Pupil
Iris
Cornea
Suspensory ligament
Vitreous humour
Ocular muscle
Optic nerve
Retinal vessels
Blind spot
Hyaloid canal
Fovea
Retina
Choroid
Sclera

The pupil is a round aperture located at the center of the iris. The iris muscles dilate and constrict the pupil in response to the amount of light. Various drugs and specific physiological and psychological states can also influence the size and the shape of the pupil.

Eye color is the result of the amount of pigment in the iris. Eye color can range from pale blue to dark brown.

Note: Keen students of iridology should read up on anatomy, physiology, and pathology to broaden their knowledge of the eye's structure and function and of diseases in general.

TOOLS FOR EYE EXAMINATION

The principal tools required for examining the eye are a magnifying glass that magnifies 8x or 10x and a flashlight that can illuminate the iris with a focused beam. I recommend a penlight with a small bulb that will not overheat the eye but lights up the iris well. It is important that the eye be illuminated from the side and that the flashlight is not aimed directly into the pupil. (Note: halogen flashlights can cause damage to eye tissue and should not be used.) If you require more sophisticated tools, you can purchase the types of instruments used by optometrists or ophthalmologists, but you can certainly do an excellent job with these simple tools.

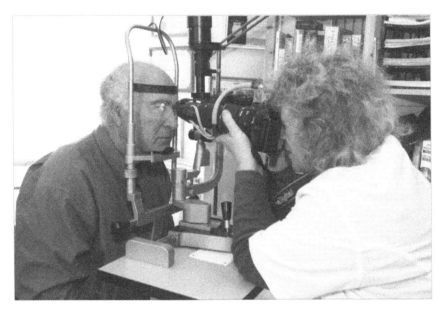

Photographing the eye

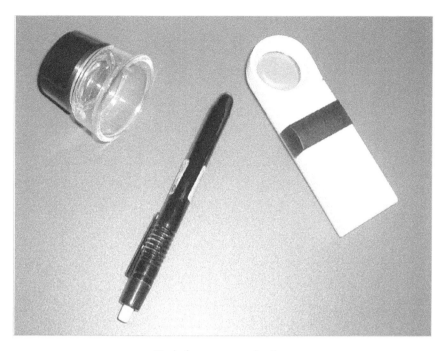

Tools for eye examination

STROMA: THE STRUCTURE OF THE FIBERS OF THE IRIS

The iris tissue is composed of weblike fibers radiating like threads outward from the center of the eye, the pupil. These fibers form the body of the iris. The markings that will be discussed later appear in and above the body of the iris. The density of these fibers—the stroma—indicates the body's strength and immunity to disease. The fiber color results from the pigment density and ranges from light blue to dark brown and all shades in between.

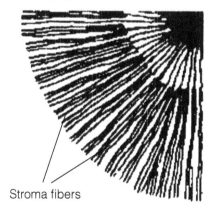

Stroma fibers

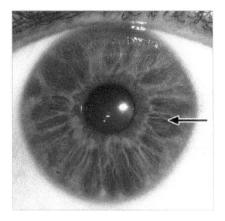
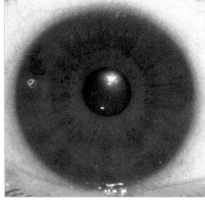

Stroma in a blue eye   Stroma in a brown eye

TRANSVERSE: FIBERS THAT CROSS THE STROMA

1. Transverse—A white fiber in the stroma that crosses the normal radial structure of the stroma. This indicates acute inflammation.

2. A red fiber that crosses the stroma indicates a blood vessel problem in that area as well as progressive inflammation.

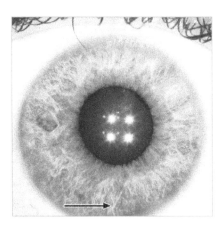
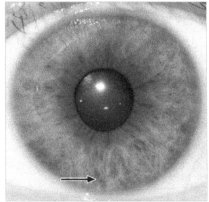

White Transverse fiber—   Red Transverse fiber—
the kidney area   blood vessels problem

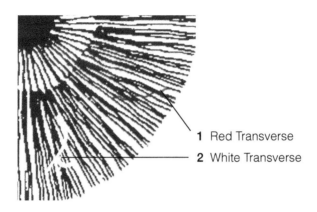

1 Red Transverse
2 White Transverse

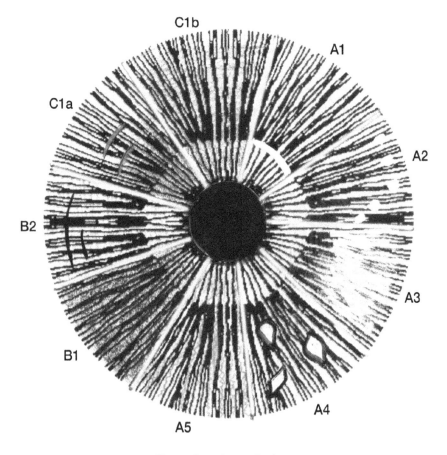

Illustration of constitutions

CHAPTER TWO

The Constitutions*

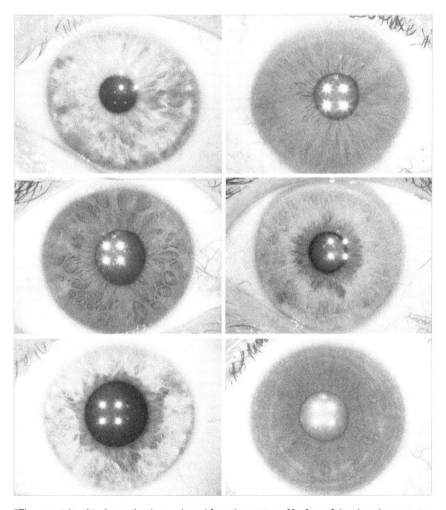

*The material in this chapter has been adapted from the writings of Professor Schmidt with permission.

The term "constitution" refers to the characteristics of the congenital structure. Genetic predispositions can remain dormant for a lifetime or can be triggered by emotional, behavioral, or environmental causes at any stage in life. A knowledge of these characteristics are essential. According to Professor Schmidt's method, all human eyes have three basic colors: blue eyes, brown eyes, and mixed eyes.

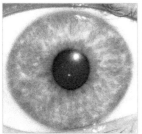 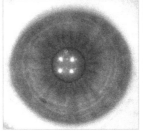 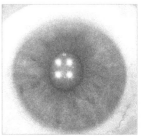

A. Blue eyes   B. Brown eyes   C. Mixed eyes (part blue and part brown)

DESCRIPTION OF THE CONSTITUTIONS

The blue-eyed group (A) is characterized by a weak lymphatic system and is called the Lymphatic Group. The brown-eyed group (B) is characterized by blood quality and blood vessel disorders and is called the Haematogenic Group. The mixed-eye group (C) is characterized by blood and lymph problems and is called the Mixed Group. Each group is divided into subgroups as illustrated in the following table:

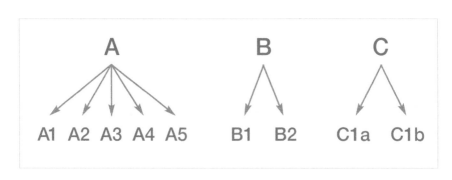

A. THE LYMPHATIC GROUP

TYPE	IDENTIFYING MARKINGS IN THE EYE
A1—Pure Lymphatic Type	A white shoelace-like ring located in the central lymphatic ring area
A2—Hydrogenoidic Type	"Tophi"—small wool-like patches
A3—Uric Acid Diathesis	Cloudiness
A4—Connective Tissue Weakness	Lacunae
A5—Neurogenic Type	"Maubach hairs"* (curly hair stroma)

B. THE HAEMATOGENIC GROUP

TYPE	IDENTIFYING MARKINGS IN THE EYE
B1—Pure Haematogenic Type	Velvety stroma
B2—Haematogenic and Tetanic Type with contraction furrows	Brown eye with contraction furrows

C. THE MIXED GROUP

TYPE	IDENTIFYING MARKINGS IN THE EYE
C1a—Type consists of one-third haematogenic and two-thirds lymphatic characteristics; mixed constitution	Tendency to green eye color with yellow-brown tints
C1b—type consists of two-thirds haematogenic and one-third lymphatic characteristics; mixed constitution	Brown eye with blue/green rim

*Maubach is the name of the Iridologist who discovered the pattern of the "curly hair" stroma.

Possible Combinations of Types

A1 +A2 +A3 + A4	**A5** + A2 + A3
A2 + A3 + A4	**B1** + A3 + A4
A3 + A2 + A4	**B2** + A2 + A3 + A4
A4 can be part of any constitution	**C1a** + A2 + A3 + A4
	C1b + A2 + A3 + A4

A—THE LYMPHATIC GROUP

A1— Pure Lymphatic Type

A clear, blue eye with a white, 2-mm-wide shoelace-like ring, surrounding the central lymph area. This location represents the intestinal ring and the nervous system ring (collarette) (see page 53). This "white shoelace" reflects the condition of these three systems.

The white ring is prominent and forms a complete circle. The ring is congenitally white and indicates lymphatic disorders. If these disorders worsen, the ring changes color from yellow to light brown, depending on the severity of the condition. This color change indicates toxin secretion.

The eye fiber structure (stroma) resembles slightly curly hairs (similar to A5).

Type A1 has a tendency toward lymphatic weakness. The lymph system is constantly "on alert." Blood tests show a level of lymphocytes/white blood cells, 50 percent higher than normal. This indicates an infection, the location of which tests are unable to pinpoint.

Predispositions of A1

- Diseases of gastric and intestinal mucosa
- Bladder infections
- Allergy to penicillin

- Allergies in general

- Sensitivity of the esophagus

- Sensitivity of the kidneys

- Sensitivity of genital mucosa

- Diseases of upper respiratory mucosa

- Tonsillitis, ENT (ear, nose, and throat) disorders

- Damaged pleura (occasionally)

This type is impatient and never satisfied. They have an apparent inability to concentrate on studies, combined with reluctance and nastiness. Children demand a lot of attention, especially when ill. (Bach Flower Remedy—Chicory can be suitable.) This type cries a lot and likes to be surrounded by people.

Important: This type is sensitive to procaine (a penicillin component). This can create a vicious circle: hidden infections are apparent; the doctor prescribes penicillin, which is likely to aggravate the symptoms due to sensitivity. Attention should be given to finding suitable medication. In addition, multivitamins should not be prescribed due to A1 type's sensitivity to their components.

Note: This is a very rare type.

How to Improve Quality of Life

- Avoid using milk and other dairy products

- Lymphatic massage and lymphatic clearing with herbs

- Maintain correct weight (to prevent stress on lymphatic system)

- Physical activity that improves lymph flow is imperative (for example, trampoline)

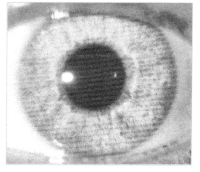

A1
(Courtesy of Professor Schmidt)

- Check and treat allergies (I use the IPEC method to neutralize allergens.)

- Always start with a minimum amount of medication and increase dosage gradually to check the body's reaction

- Eat lots of green vegetables and drink green vegetable and green-leaf juices (preferably organic)

A2—Hydrogenoidic Type

A blue eye with small cotton wool-like yellow or white patches called "tophi." Tophi are located adjacent to the cilliary border and near the collarette.

In a blue eye, the tophi should be white, but deterioration of the lymph system can cause the tophi to turn yellowish to brown.

In a brown eye, the tophi are yellow (see Mixed Group on page 40).

A large amount of tophi in an eye indicates a person who has been suffering from weakness of constitution for some time. If there is only a single tophi, its location should be noted.

Tophi are generally located homogenously around the external rim of the iris and/or slightly toward the center. Single white patches or groups, similar to tophi, can be found randomly in the iris. This indicates arsenic poisoning.

Type A2 belongs primarily to the Lymphatic Group and therefore suffers from lymphatic sensitivity. Being a Hydrogenoidic Type, in addition to belonging to the lymphatic group, causes disorders of the water-management system—kidneys, urinary tract, and bladder. This type will suffer from lymph system and lymph fluid disorders, perspiration, and salivary problems as well.

Predispositions of A2

- Colds

- Asthma

- Allergies

- Kidney weakness

- Rheumatic aches and pains in the small joints

- Dizziness

- Loss of balance

- Buzzing in the ears

- Sensitive sinuses

- Dental problems from childhood

- Shoulder pain caused by dental problems (inflammation of a tooth nerve can cause pain that radiates to the shoulder)

- Scurf rim—twin of type A3 (both suffer from similar disorders)

- Rash—urticaria (hives)

- Eczema and other skin disorders

- Problems with the water-management system and bodily fluids

- Tendency toward anemia

- Tendency toward fear and a great worrier

One tophi is enough to define a person as A2. The more tophi present in the eye, the more severe the typical A2 complaints will be. A2 types have inherited toxins that cause the kidneys to over-work and consequently weaken them. The markings indicating these toxins—the tophi—will not disappear even after the disorders have been treated.

The person will suffer from bone pain when the tophi are closer to the cilliary border. (See Iridology Chart.) The person will suffer from muscular pain when the tophi are closer to the collarette. (See Iridology Chart).

In most cases, a white marking can be observed in the lung and pleura area of the iris, indicating a family history of tuberculosis.

IMPORTANT NOTE

It is not a given that any type will suffer from all listed complaints; most people only suffer from some of them, depending on their lifestyle. The better care they take of themselves—nutrition, drinking correctly, sleep, balanced emotional life—the fewer symptoms they will have. The more a person ignores his/her own needs, the worse the symptoms will be.

How to Improve Quality of Life

- Use herbs to strengthen the kidneys

- Reflexology—two cycles of eight to ten sessions per year

- Warm the kidneys with ginger compresses

- Moxa treatments from a qualified therapist. Moxa is a cigar made of Artimisia Vulgaris, a leaf from Japan with many curing properties, used to heat the place of the ailment.

- Eat organic food—preferably macrobiotic

- Avoid preserved food and reduce salt intake significantly to prevent edema

- Avoid eating corn, wheat, white flour, oranges, high-fat cheese, animal protein, cold food, and beverages that can damage the kidneys (See details of allergy-causing foods on page 129.)

- Drink correctly

- Adzuki beans are recommended for strengthening the kidneys (most effective to consume the beans and their cooking water)

*"Anything that lengthens a product's shelf life,
shortens the time spent on earth."*

—S.B., A VERY WISE STUDENT OF MINE

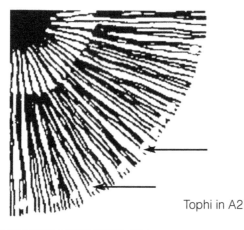

Tophi in A2

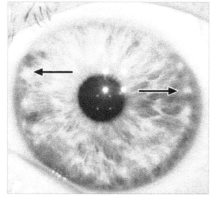

A2+A4

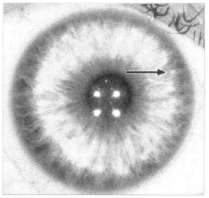

A2+A4

A3—Uric Acid Diathesis

In blue eyes, the iris will be partially or mostly covered with a deposit of white or gray cloudiness, starting at the collarette and extending toward the cilliary border, or vice-versa, hiding the signs underneath on the iris. In a brown iris, the cloud will appear gray to yellowish or light brown in color.

The most common characteristic of this type is no sense of thirst.

Predispositions of A3

- Rheumatic aches and pains, mainly in large joints
- Kidney weakness and tendency to produce kidney stones

- Gout

- Uric acid values in blood tests are higher than normal due to a genetic metabolic defect; in most cases, there are high uric acid values (over 6 mg/dl. Normal levels are 2.5–4.5 mg/dl)

- Middle ear disorders (In Chinese medicine the kidneys are energetically parallel to the ears and the knees. They are all located on the same meridian.)

- Dry skin

- Hair loss

- Scurf rim = twin of type A2

- Tendency toward edema, swollen arms, legs, and face due to water-management system disorders

- Knee problems

- Ringing and tingling in the ears (due to disorders of ear-fluid management)

- Changes in blood pressure

- Tendency to have bags under the eyes due to kidney weakness

- Tendency to anemia

- Lacks initiative, finds executing ideas difficult, and tends to procrastinate

Type A3 is trapped in a vicious circle: on one hand, weak kidneys and the tendency to produce kidney stones, and, on the other hand, a tendency not to drink enough due to the absence of a sense of thirst. This combination accelerates kidney-stone production unless the individual is taught how often to drink and drinks out of self-awareness.

Creating a positive health change in A3 types is the easiest. Even though the predisposition is genetic, health improvement or deterioration depends on lifestyle.

How to Improve Quality of Life

- Avoid heavy physical strain that can weaken the kidneys and damage the heart

- Learn to drink enough water with low-sodium content; a combination of sodium and chlorine is damaging to this type

- Avoid eating salty and spicy food

- Do not drink regular black tea

- Reduce body acidity by avoiding vegetables from the nightshade family—tomatoes, eggplant, green peppers, and potatoes (Very ripe, organically grown tomatoes are permitted.)

- Avoid food containing vinegar

- Avoid meat, animal fat, and especially internal organs

- Take care not to catch cold and make sure to keep the kidney area warm

- Do not use skin creams; creams clog the pores and prevent the skin from "breathing" properly. (It is very tempting to lubricate the skin with cream, as dry skin is common in this type because of insufficient liquid intake.)

- Before showering, dry-massage the body with a natural sea sponge, starting from the periphery toward the heart

- Take dry saunas and alternating cold and hot baths

- Consider eating seaweed; consult a professional first if there are any suspected thyroid disorders

- Drink the juice of two to three freshly squeezed lemons diluted in water every day (Drink the juice through a straw to prevent harming tooth enamel.)

"The body transforms every green vegetable into blood!"
—ANONYMOUS

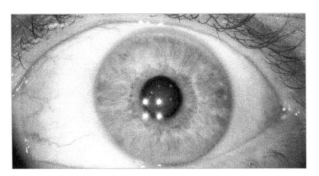

A2+A3+A4

- If predisposed anemia develops, add iron-rich foods and organic iron supplements to the diet to increase iron levels. Iron additives should be accompanied by a supplement that aids absorption (e.g., vitamin C). Recommended foods include green leaves, nuts, whole wheat, dried peas, seaweed (under nutritional advice), artichoke, fish eggs, sardines, pumpkin seeds, chickpeas, fenugreek, sunflower seeds, sesame paste (tahini), miso, wheat germ, wheat bran, soya (dried beans), dried lentils, cocoa powder, and white beans.

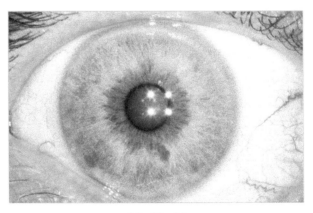

A3+A2+A4

"Dead men, of all people the most discreet, tell no tales of the doctor who has sent them to their long account."
—MOLIERE, A DOCTOR DESPITE HIMSELF

A4—Connective Tissue Weakness

This type is identified by lacunae—areas sparse in stroma fibers that look like "pools" in the tissue of the iris. An additional A4-type characteristic is widely spaced stroma fibers with various density levels. The less dense they are, the weaker the body. A kind of bordered pool is formed because of the lack and weakness of the fibers. Lacunae (lack of tissue or lake) can be seen without a magnifying glass. The various kinds of lacunae are detailed in Chapter 5.

This type is characterized by weak connective tissue: muscles, sinews, cartilage, skeleton, and supportive organs.

Note: Despite the tissue weakness, this type likes sports such as boxing and weight lifting and seems strong and hardy. This is misleading because the weakness is internal and appears at a later age.

Congenital weakness can be altered
by leading a suitable lifestyle.

Predispositions of A4

- Weakness of blood vessels and heart (veins, valves, widening of blood vessels, heart attacks)
- Varicose veins
- Internal organ prolapse—prolapse of the uterus especially after giving birth
- Intestinal prolapse (protruding stomach in men)
- Tendency to hernias
- Cystocele and weakness of the bladder
- Hemorrhoids
- Lower back pain, mainly in lumbar vertebrae
- Weakness of the legs, mainly in older people, with a tendency to "drag" a leg
- Prostate problems
- Sluggish intestines (constipation)

- Sluggish pancreas and tendency toward diabetes

- Weak immune system, tendency toward colds and tonsillitis

- Fatigue, mental weakness

- A4 children tend to be incontinent longer and start walking later than other children

- Tendency to develop neoplasm (cysts, fibroids, malignant and nonmalignant growths)

- Flatulence and gas after meals

- Formation of intestinal diverticuli that store waste and can cause chronic constipation or diarrhea; waste stored in the gut for a long period, in a humid atmosphere full of germs and parasites, may cause intestinal growths

- Difficulty falling asleep and, consequently, difficulty waking up in the morning

- An extremely sensitive type, takes too much to heart, has low self-esteem and feels inferior, anticipates, likes to help, vulnerable, and tends to cry; loves nature and the color green

Everyone who has type A4 in their constitution may have the symptoms but not everyone who has the symptoms is A4.

THE FOLLOWING RULE IS TRUE FOR ALL CONSTITUTIONS:

Do not search the eye for markings that correlate with the symptoms.
Do evaluate the symptoms by the markings found in the eye.

The more lacunae there are and the deeper and bigger they are, the greater the weakness. Most lacunae are genetic and cannot be changed. There are lacunae that are acquired through surgery, injury, or accident. When an organ or tissue is damaged, lacunae will form in that location. The color, size, and depth of the lacunae enable us to evaluate the severity of the injury.

In some cases, surgery leaves no marking on the iris. This is because anesthesia prevents a reaction from the nervous system.

Healing signs will appear in the lacunae after appropriate treatment and strengthening the body. These weblike signs indicate that the body is in the process of healing the tissues and the damaged organ.

How to Improve Quality of Life

- Avoid very strenuous physical activity and take care of the body

- Avoid white sugar (Every gram of sugar consumed takes 1 mg of calcium from the bones.)

- Do moderate physical activity followed by a massage; avoid sports that put a strain on one side of the body, such as tennis, squash, and basketball

- Avoid lifting heavy weights

- Avoid horseback riding as it can damage the spinal vertebrae

- Eat deep-sea fish

- Pay attention to nutrition—avoid big meals; do not be overweight

- Strengthen the immune system—for example, through complementary medicine, lifestyle modification, herbs, physical activity, hydrotherapy, and, above all, improving self-confidence, emotional expression, and body awareness

Note: Even if a person adheres to all the healthy lifestyle rules, chooses a diet carefully, and follows all the instructions in the naturopathy books, but nevertheless leads a stressful, pressured life, lacks love of self and others, and is unable to fulfill ambitions, he or she is likely to become ill. On the other hand, people who are surrounded by love, give and receive, lead a joyful life, fully express themselves, and fulfill their ambitions can generally eat any kind of food they like and still lead a long and healthy life.

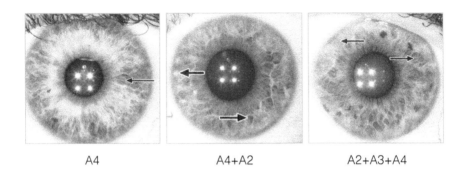

A4   A4+A2   A2+A3+A4

A5—Neurogenic Type

A blue-eyed person with dense "curly hair" stroma (Maubach hairs, named after Maubach who defined them). The curlier the fibers, the more sensitive the type.

Very dense areas of the iris covered with white indicate a local irritation or infection. This is generally observed in the lung area, genital area, and bladder.

Contraction furrows are common in A5s and indicate high stress levels and a tendency toward headaches. For additional information on contraction furrows, see Chapter 12.

This type is physically strong but has weak nerves.

Predispositions of A5

- Nervous disorders, particularly in the central nervous system

- Headaches/migraines caused by stress and blood-flow obstructions to the neck area

- Nausea and pressure in the head without a migraine

- Constriction of blood vessels in the skull area

- Urinary tract infections

- Frequent urination due to stress

- Tendency to develop Alzheimer disease, Parkinson's disease, or paralysis in old age

- Critical, responsible, hardworking, perfectionist; they exhaust themselves through overexertion that can lead to a nervous breakdown; love justice; impatient—fear inability to reach targets on time; get angry, women tend to be hysterical, men less

Note: Everything is genetically predisposed, but if a suitable lifestyle is adhered to, most of the tendencies will remain dormant.

> *"The only thing we have to fear is the fear itself!"*
> —FRANKLIN DELANO ROOSEVELT

How to Improve Quality of Life

- Macrobiotic nutrition (70 percent minimum)

- Avoid foods containing chemicals

- Avoid hard cheese, sausage, and preserved foods

- Herbs

- Homeopathy

- Schuessler's salts (prescribed by a qualified therapist)

- Yoga

- Meditation and relaxation

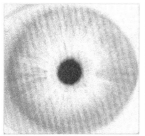 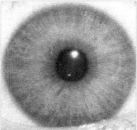 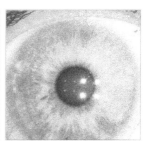

| A5 | A5 | A5 with A2+A4 |

B—THE HAEMATOGENIC GROUP

B1—Pure Haematogenic Type

This type is extremely uncommon. Schmidt defined the term from *haema* meaning "blood" combined with *genic* meaning "created." This type's pathology deals with blood disorders and dyscrasia—combination of blood and bodily fluids.

This dark-brown eye is characterized by smooth, velvety-like stroma with no contraction furrows. Occasionally, congestion will appear on the iris—hill-like mounds that indicate high stress levels. (Congestion can appear in B2s, in addition to other markings, and indicates an increase in stress levels.)

The iris is smooth with no other markings. Lacunae can be present.

Occasionally, pale surfaces that appear to have been sanded down can be seen. This indicates a local irritation of a specific organ or system, or a lack of certain minerals, mainly magnesium and zinc.

A B1's body temperature does not rise when ill. The body's lack of response to disease is due to a lack of basic minerals. Therefore, a supplement of iodine, copper, iron, and gold should be considered.

This type suffers from problems with blood flow and gland secretion. Lymphocyte levels are normal, compared to the lymphatic type who shows a marked increase in lymphocyte levels.

Predispositions of B1

- Lymphosarcoma-lymphopenia
- Hodgkin's and non-Hodgkin's disease
- Lymphoblastoma
- Sarcoma
- Leukemia
- Uterine cancer in woman
- Prostate cancer in men
- Tendency to anemia

Note: Disease in type B1 breaks out quickly and lethally.

In my clinical work I have only come across two people who were B1s in fifteen years. One was an unmarried forty-year-old woman who wanted to have a baby and discovered large, bleeding fibroids in her uterus and was about to have urgent surgery. The other was her sister who had the same constitution and passed away after a hysterectomy due to malignant tumors that were not discovered in time. When the forty-year-old went through the Iris diagnosis, she was planning to have a baby, but the doctors wanted to remove her uterus to prevent future problems. They mentioned also the possibility of removing only the fibroids without any guarantee as to what would occur next, and she came to me to ask for my advice. According to the tendency of the B1 constitution to suddenly develop malignancy, I explained to her the decision I would make if I were in her situation. Considering her age and her desire to have a baby, I would at first remove the fibroids, and, if everything goes smoothly, try to get pregnant and, immediately after the birth, have the uterus removed.

How to Improve Quality of Life

- Correct nutrition
- Avoid dairy products, which can damage the lymphatic system (immune system)
- Supplements to replace lacking minerals
- Ongoing medical supervision and regular checkups—breast and uterus in woman, prostate in men, particularly after the fertile years

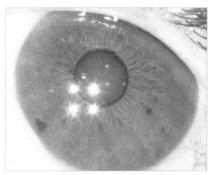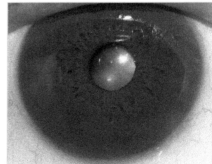

B1

"The only fixed thing in the universe is change."
—ALBERT EINSTEIN

B2—Tetanic Type with Contraction Furrows

This is a brown eye with contraction furrows (see page 111). A single furrow is enough to categorize this type.

Predispositions of B2

- Psychosomatic illness
- Women tend to have hypothyroidism (hyperthyroidism in some cases)
- Parathyroid function disorders
- Muscular contractions in hip and stomach, stomachache
- Tendency to angina pectoris in later years
- Migraines
- Contractions of respiratory system
- Dizziness and ringing in the ears
- Faintness (consciousness is not lost in most cases)
- Cry easily and tendency to hysteria, mainly in woman (similar to A5)
- Depressive tendency
- Disorders in glycemia management—mainly hypoglycemia that causes a drop in energy and sleepiness during the day
- Tendency toward diabetes
- Fear of death and the unknown
- Claustrophobia, fear of heights
- Fear of disease

- Fear of exams, finds self-expression difficult

- Choking sensation—dislikes wearing ties

- Feels cold and tingling in fingers and feet

- Muscle contraction in legs

- Sensation of pressure in the chest (mainly due to gas, resulting from unsuitable eating habits)

- Rapid pulse, variations in pulse

- Long and difficult first labor in woman

- Intelligent, empathetic

- Suspicious

- Likes spicy food

Note: A person does not necessarily have all the symptoms. In most cases, only some of the symptoms appear, although some people do have all the symptoms.

How to Improve Quality of Life

- B2s should be taught to communicate and improve personal relations

- Pursue a creative and/or artistic occupation

- Practice self-expression and public speaking

- Suitable nutrition

- Mineral supplements (calcium and potassium prescribed by a qualified therapist)

- Schuessler's salts (prescribed by a qualified therapist)

- Bach remedies—rescue remedy plus mimulus

- Psychotherapy, spiritual awareness, and emotional work

Treatments can minimize the symptoms.

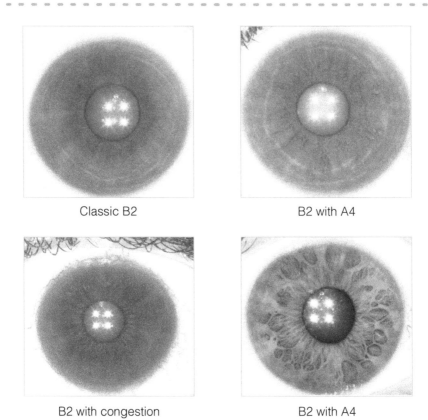

| Classic B2 | B2 with A4 |

| B2 with congestion | B2 with A4 |

C—THE MIXED GROUP

C1a—One-Third Haematogenic and Two-Thirds Lymphatic Characteristics

The same proportions are apparent in the eye and in the disorders from which this type suffers. The brown portion of the eye includes B2's thyroid disorder and the blue portion consists of A2 plus A5's iris markings and constitutional weaknesses.

The mixed eye has a greenish color tinged with brown (proportions are not symmetrical). The brown portion is closer to the pupil and starts at the collarette. The lighter portion is next to the cilliary border.

Mixed-group eyes appear to be brown, but closer inspection through a magnifying glass reveals leaflike layers colored yellow, green, and brown.

Changes in the iris color take place from the lymphatic constitution to the haematogenic. This is the reason that the prominent upper layer is brown. It is very important to differentiate between C1a and C1b types.

C1a's main weaknesses are in the liver, gall bladder, and pancreas. The majority of disorders will be in these organs. This type suffers from a constant lack of digestive enzymes.

Most eyes of this type have contraction furrows that indicate stress levels, anxiety, and fear (from type B2).

Predispositions of C1a

- Angina pectoris
- Pressure on the heart due to gas (Roemheld syndrome)
- Tendency to diabetes mellitus
- Thyroid disorders
- Anxiety and fear that affect the heart and, in turn, the thyroid
- Tendency to produce gallstones (by the time most clients of this type come for diagnosis, their gallbladders have already been removed)
- Fast eating that tires the digestive system
- Rapid pulse, irregular heartbeat
- Tendency toward heart disease, varicose veins, and hemorrhoids

How to Improve Quality of Life

- Suitable nutrition—avoiding fatty, fried, and sweet foods
- Need to be taught to eat correctly—to eat slowly, chew each mouthful well, and eat small, frequent meals
- Herbs

- Emotional processing for clearing resentment and anger—typical emotions in people with gallbladder and liver weakness (Chinese medicine)

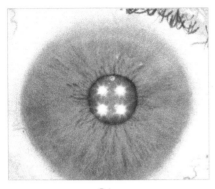
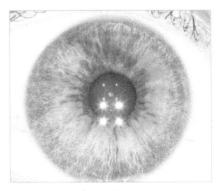

C1a   C1a with A4

C1b—Two-Thirds Haematogenic and One-Third Lymphatic Characteristics

This is a light brown eye, slightly green-gray and dull. The brown portion is closer to the pupil and starts at the collarette. The lighter portion is adjacent to the cilliary border. This type's main disorder is iron absorption.

Predispositions of C1b

- Deficient iron absorption; constant lack of iron that affects the heart and weakens the thyroid

- Disorders associated with C1a and B2

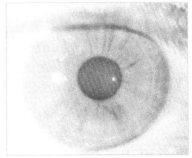

C1b
(Courtesy of Professor Schmidt)

How to Improve Quality of Life

- Make sure to eat a naturally iron-rich diet and to take supplements to improve iron absorption

- All recommendations associated with B2 and C1a

PART TWO

Markings
in the Iris

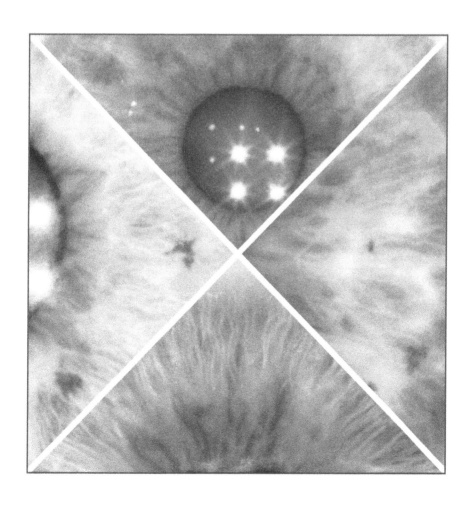

CHAPTER 3

· · · · · ·

Divisions of the Iris

The pupil (pupilla) is the center of the iris.

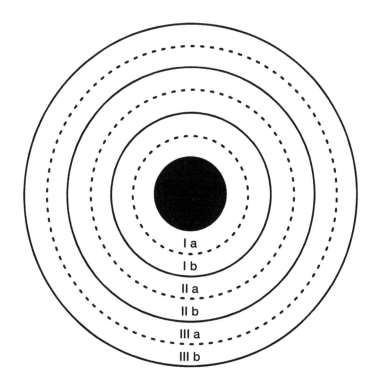

Area I

Reflects organs for processing and absorbing substances.

I a. Stomach

I b. Intestine (the collarette); this area represents the central
lymphatic area and the autonomic nervous system

Area II

Reflects organs that transfer and utilize substances.

II a. Blood and blood vessels

II b. Muscular system, heart, kidneys, adrenal glands,
pancreas, and gallbladder

Area III

Reflects organs that support the body, secretion organs,
and organs of toxin elimination.

III a. Bones/skeleton

III b. Skin

Secretion of toxins: liver, spleen

Secretion in general: skin, mucosa of mouth and nose,
urethra, and rectum

CHAPTER 4

The Digestive System

THE STOMACH

The stomach area is the area adjacent to the pupil. It resembles a smooth-textured ring of uniform width (1 mm) surrounding the pupil. The colors and texture of this area reflect the biochemical state of the stomach.

A stomach area that resembles a white aura indicates an overly acidic stomach. A gray stomach area indicates an overly alkaline stomach. Neither of these states is desirable, and an immediate dietary change is necessary to regain gastric balance. The relationship between two groups of minerals determines if foods are acid or alkaline. Metallic minerals—for example calcium, magnesium, potassium, sodium, and iron—become alkaline when reacting with oxygen. Nonmetallic minerals, such as phosphorus, chlorine, and sulfur, create acids.

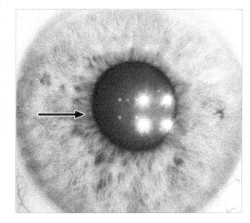

The stomach area

Foods that create an acidic reaction:

Artichoke	Chocolate	Lentils	Sauerkraut
Asparagus	Cocoa	Meat	Seeds
Beer	Coffee	Mushrooms	Semolina
Brussels sprouts	Dried beans	Nuts	Spinach
Buckwheat	Eggs	Oats	Tea
Chard	Fish	Olives	Wheat and wheat products
Cheese	Gherkins	Peanuts	White Sugar
Chicken	Horseradish	Plums	Wine
	Legumes	Rice	

Foods that create an alkaline reaction:

Almonds	Citrus fruit	Melon	Sabra fruit
Aubergine	Corn flour	Mulberries	Sesame
Avocado	Custard apple	Okra	Sprouted legumes
Bananas	Dates	Papaya	Sweet corn
Beetroot	Figs	Parsley	Sweet potato
Broccoli	Grapes	Peaches	Tahini
Cabbage	Green peas	Persimmon	Tomatoes
Carrots	Guava	Pomegranate	Turnip
Cauliflower	Kohlrabi	Potatoes	Watermelon
Celery	Lettuce	Pumpkin	
Cherries	Mango	Red pepper	

"Treating a disease after it has appeared
is like digging a well when you're thirsty."
—CHINESE SAYING

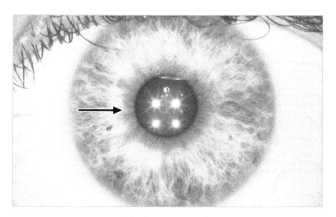

Alkaline stomach

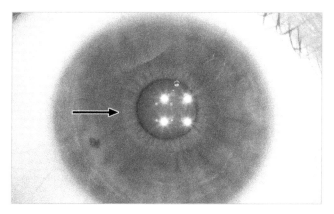

Acidic stomach in brown eye

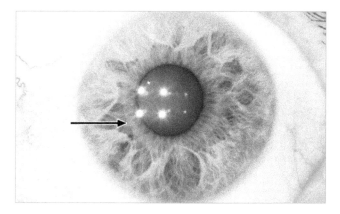

Acidic stomach in blue eye

Additional markings in stomach area:

- Lacunae in the stomach area indicate gastric weakness.

- Black lacunae in the stomach area indicate candida. The darker the color and the larger the area covered, the more active the candida. This finding can be verified by checking the white of the eye. (See illustrations.)

- Pigments (see page 103).

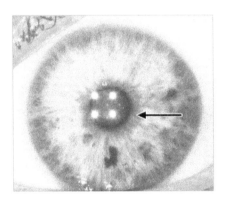 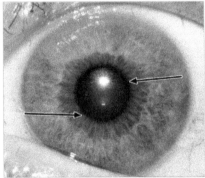

Candida

"A journey of a thousand miles
must begin with a single step."

—LAO TZU

THE INTESTINES

The ring surrounding the stomach area reflects the state of the small and large intestine. This area represents all of the following: 1) Intestinal border, 2) Central lymphatic system, 3) Autonomic nervous system, 4) Spinal nerves, and 5) "Time Risk" (as researched by the Italian iridologist, Dr. Daniele De Lo Rito.)

The abdomen and the intestine are the body's "furnace." If the "furnace" goes out or is not properly fed, the entire body suffers. Physical intestinal disorders affect an individual's emotions, thoughts, and intellect.

Chinese medicine calls this area the "hara" and regards it as an additional heart. Apparently, there is logic in the expression "gut feeling" or "having the guts." In Chinese medicine, the colon's twin organs are the lungs. The lungs feed the body with essential oxygen, which is equally important for intestinal functioning. A "blocked" lung or a "blocked" colon blocks the life flow through the body. If either does not function properly, death will result. Therefore, it is imperative to keep the colon clean and regular.

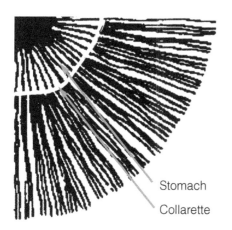

Stomach

Collarette

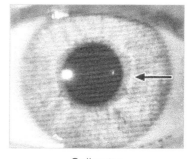

Collarette

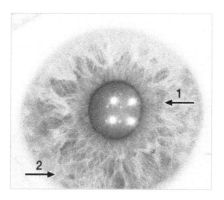

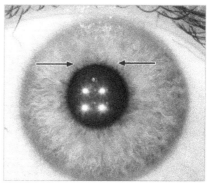

1 Atrophied collarette (intestine)
2 Ballooned intestine

Strictured intestine

Eighty percent of colon cancer tumors are located in the areas indicated in the illustration at right.

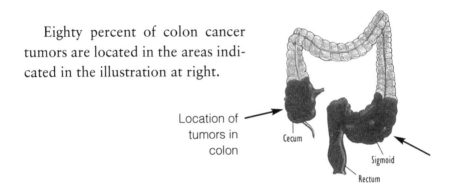

Location of tumors in colon

Cecum

Sigmoid

Rectum

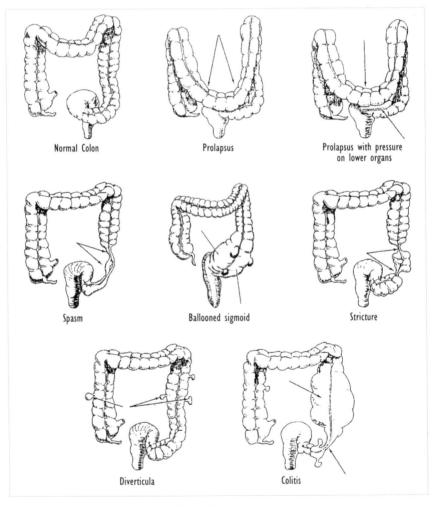

Normal Colon

Prolapsus

Prolapsus with pressure on lower organs

Spasm

Ballooned sigmoid

Stricture

Diverticula

Colitis

Colon Pathology

Images 1 through 8 of the colon used courtesy of Dr. David J. Pesek.

Collarette—Intestinal Border

The collarette is a reflection in the iris of the body's actual intestinal structure:

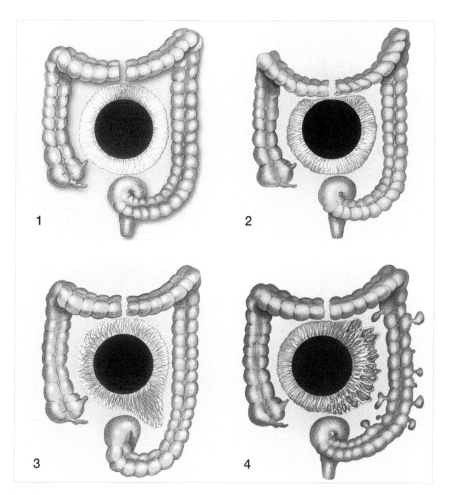

LEGEND

1 Normal, healthy colon

2 Prolapse of transverse colon

3 Prolapse of sigmoid

4 Diverticula in descending colon

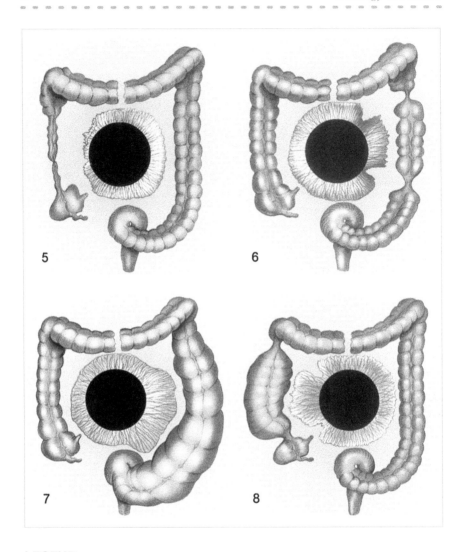

LEGEND

5 Stricture of ascending colon

6 Strictures in descending colon

7 Ballooning of descending colon

8 Colitis in ascending colon

Central Lymphatic System (Overlaying the Collarette)

The lymphatic system is part of the body's immune system. The immune system identifies "intruders" and destroys them. When the body is overloaded with toxins, the immune system is unable to keep up the pace, the "intruders" gain control, and illness results.

- Toxins—molecules that comprise a substance—parasites, emotions, and thoughts

- Substances—food, beverages, medications, supplements, narcotics, tobacco smoke, atmospheric factors that are detrimental to the body

- Parasites—bacteria, parasites, fungi, mold, and viruses

- Emotions—over- or underexpression of anger, rage, resentment, jealousy, and hatred

- Thoughts—worrying, pessimistic, suicidal thoughts

In a healthy eye, the collarette area will be the natural iris color. Any change in color or tissue structure indicates a change in one of the four systems reflected in this area and according to Daniele De Lo Rito, a turning point in the individual's life.

White indicates inflammation, phlegm, and irritation. White in the collarette area indicates rheumatic acid. The body is unable to rid itself of excess acidity. Acidity causes rheumatic pain, phlegm production, restlessness, anxiety, hyperactivity of most organs, and fast metabolism, particularly of the thyroid.

People with these symptoms have difficulty in relationships, are hard to live with, and are overly irritable.

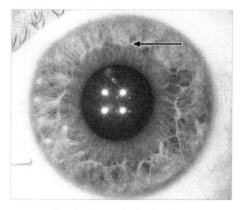

Central Lymphatic System

Autonomic Nervous System (Overlaying the Collarette)

A symmetrical collarette indicates a balanced nervous system. A broken collarette indicates a weak nervous system. The more the intestine droops to the sides, the more prone the person is to mental breakdown and life crises. Nervous weakness—mental breakdown.

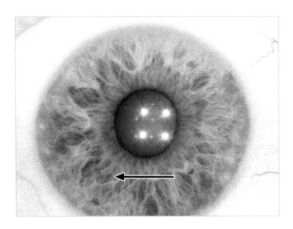

Atrophy of the nervous system border—weak nerves

A missing collarette (atrophy) indicates:

1. A weak intestine

2. Weak nerves and difficulty dealing with traumatic events

3. Sensitive vertebrae in the atrophied area (see page 57)

4. A turning point in life during emotional distress

Atrophy of the nervous system border—weak nerves

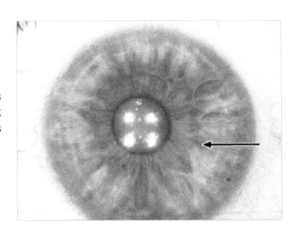

Spinal Vertebrae Nerves (Overlaying the Collarette)

According to Dr. Jensen, the spine is reflected in the iris in two areas:

1. In the iridology chart between 7:30 and 8:30

2. In the collarette as follows:

   - Between 11:00 and 1:00—cervical nerves

   - Between 01:00 and 05:00—thoracic nerves

   - Between 05:00 and 08:00—lumbar nerves

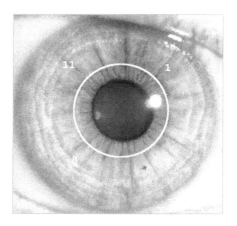

Location of spinal nerves on the collarette

The above information gives us an accurate evaluation of two spinal aspects:

1. Structure of vertebrae

2. The influence the functioning of the vertebral nerves has on the internal organs (chiropractic)

CHAPTER 5

* * * * * *

Lacunae

Lacunae are round to oval-shaped formations that appear on the stroma and are characterized by shape, color, depth, size, and location. Lacunae indicate organic weakness of the connective tissue. The weakness of the iris tissue where the lacunae are situated reflects structural weakness of an organ or of a complete system of connective tissue in the body.

Lacunae in the intestinal area do not indicate type A4. They only indicate intestinal weakness. Black lacunae in the intestinal area indicate: 1) worms, 2) microorganisms (candida), and 3) intestinal weakness, sluggish peristaltic motion, and accumulation of toxins and refuse.

Note: Most lacunae are congenital, but some are acquired through organ damage caused by surgery, accident, change in organ function, and so on. The lacunae's appearance, size, and color indicate the severity of the damage to the organ or the complete system.

THE STRUCTURE OF THE LACUNAE

The iris is composed of four layers of tissue. The lacunae's depth indicates the following:

1. The upper layer, colored like the iris, reflects genetic, congenital weakness.

2. The second, white, layer reflects an acute/inflamed state.

3. The third, gray, layer reflects a subacute, chronic state.

4. The fourth and deepest layer, black, reflects an atrophied state.

The deeper the lacunae, the weaker the organ. Occasionally, lacunae can reflect a combination of two states: part of the organ can be in an acute state, and another part of the same organ can be atrophied.

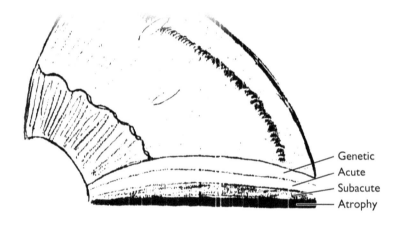

The four layers of the iris

HOW TO INTERPRET LACUNAE

- If a single lacuna is present, refer to the specific organ as located on the iridology chart.

- A large number of lacunae in both eyes indicate a general weakness of connective tissue.

- A large number of lacunae in the head area reflect weakness there (memory problems, learning disabilities, thoughts, and so on).

- A large number of lacunae in the leg area reflect leg weakness (standing, walking, paresthesia [tingling]).

- A large number of lacunae in one eye and few or none in the other eye reflect weakness of one side of the body.

- Lacunae in the intestinal area reflect dysfunction and weakness of the intestine.

Note: A large number of lacunae only in the intestinal area do not indicate a type A4.

- The greater the number of lacunae, the greater the weakness.

- The darker the lacunae, the greater the damage to the organ.

- Pay special attention to lacunae in the heart, pancreas, and liver.

TYPES OF LACUNAE

Closed Lacunae—Genetic, have clear boundaries, and are the same color as the iris. Even though this type of lacunae is genetic, they can become activate during states of extreme weakness and lack of vitality.

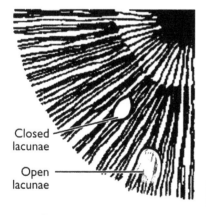

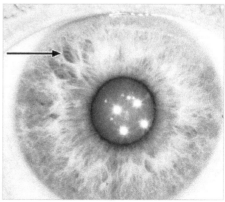

Closed and open launae　　　　　Closed lacunae in blue eye

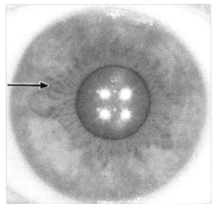 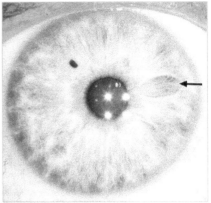

Closed lacunae

Open Lacunae—The closed end of the lacunae is adjacent to the collarette. The open end faces the cilliary border. Open lacunae indicate an unfinished process and immediate risk to the organ. It also indicates a decrease in vitality—for example, open lacunae in the heart area can indicate approaching acute heart failure, and open lacunae in the head area can indicate an approaching stroke. *Knowledge of sclerology is beneficial, as markings in the white of the eye can accurately indicate the urgency of these states. (See Chapter 14.)*

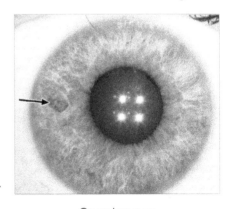

Open lacunae

Crypt—A diamond-shaped lacunae indicates chronic damage to an organ. The deeper and darker the lacunae, the greater the damage. White markings and red lines in a crypt indicate an acute attack with functional blood vessel failure. White crypt lacunae in the stomach area indicate an ulcer. A black crypt in the pancreas area indicates a cyst and risk of necrosis of the organ.

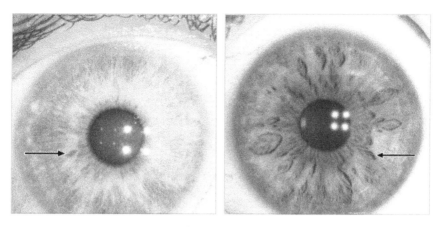

Crypt lacunae

Honeycomb/Waben—These are lacunae that resemble a cluster of small, connected circles, similar to a honeycomb. These lacunae indicate organ weakness due to unsuitable nutrition, lacking in vital substances. Waben in the lung area indicate cirrhosis. Waben in the pancreas area indicate pancreatic dysfunction.

Note: A dark to black color indicates atrophy of an organ.

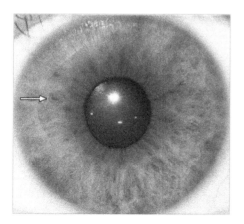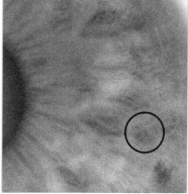

Honeycomb/Waben

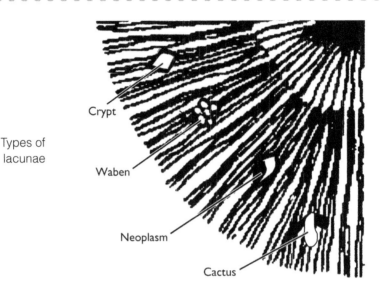

Types of
lacunae

Crypt

Waben

Neoplasm

Cactus

Neoplasm—Part of the lacunae are white, indicating an acute state; part are black, indicating partial atrophy. These lacunae indicate a severe state—development of benign or malignant cells.

Cactus—These are lacunae composed of three parts, similar to cactus leaves. These lacunae indicate the possibility of a benign or malignant tumor. Verifying the markings in the sclera is crucial to determining current pathology.

Steps—Lacunae shaped like a step. The number of steps joined together indicates the severity of a problem. This indicates development of a malignant or benign tumor.

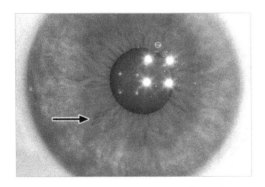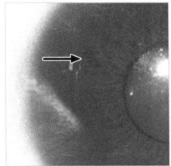

Steps lacunae

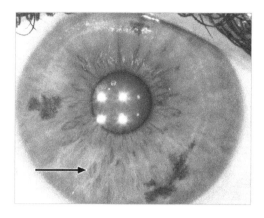

Steps lacunae

Torpedo—Indicates an advanced stage of tumor development. The root of the torpedo indicates the tumor's source. The direction of its development indicates the location of secondary growths.

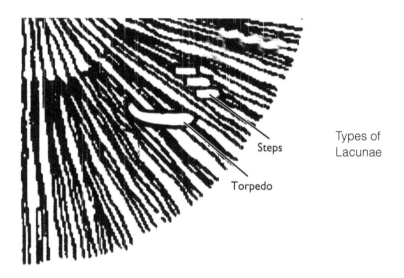

Steps

Torpedo

Types of
Lacunae

Beait—These lacunae indicate the beginning of a malignant tumor.

Asparagus—Asparagus lacunae in the testicle area indicate cysts. Asparagus lacunae in the head area indicate memory loss, pituitary dysfunction, microdenoma, prolactinoma, pinealoma, and overstimulation of the hypothalamus. (John Andrew, Ireland 2006). It may also indicate development of a malignant tumor. (Professor Schmidt).

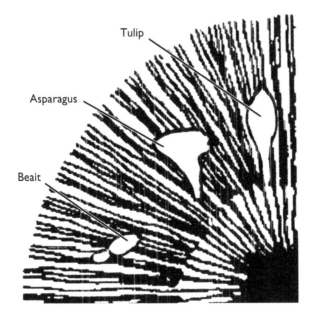

Tulip

Asparagus

Beait

Types of
Lacunae

"How do people know if a particular herb is good for them?
When they are drawn to it as a man to his love, as a baby
to its mother's breast, as man believes in his God."

—AVI YAACOBOVITZ, HERBALIST

Tulip—These types of lacunae are specific to the head area. They have a one-pointed end, similar to a tulip. They indicate a disorder of the hypophysis (pituitary gland) and severe brain damage. If the lacunae are deeper than the first three layers of stroma, it indicates depression and mental disorders from insanity and psychosis to schizophrenia. Marks in the iris indicating a head injury can also indicate leg problems.

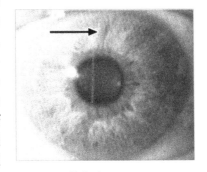

Tulip lacunae
(Courtesy of Professor Schmidt)

OBSERVATIONS FROM MY CLINICAL EXPERIENCE

Not every tumor developing in the body will be seen in the iris; however, if markings do appear in the eye, pathological developments will be present in the body. Reliable information cannot be retrieved by an amateur glance at the eye. A professional iridologist should be consulted, and, even then, it is important to keep in mind that not all genetic tendencies are activated in the body. Construct a complete picture by combining additional data retrieved from the iris and preferably from the sclera. This avoids any unnecessary distress resulting from receiving inaccurate information on the clients' behalf. I believe the importance of iridology lies in this method's ability to save lives by giving advance warning about a severe disorder early enough to be able to treat it.

CHAPTER 6

⊛ ⊛ ⊛ ⊛ ⊛ ⊛

Intoxification

The iris markings indicating intoxification—the physiological state produced by a poison or other toxic substance—resemble a sun with symmetrical rays originating from the pupillary border (the gastric area) and terminating near the outer rim of the iris. (In comparison to C1a, in which the brown portion of the eye is not symmetrical.)

Reddish-brown intoxification indicates autointoxification caused by chemical substances entering the body by mouth, through radiation, injection, or inhalation from the following sources:

- Foods contaminated by pesticides (weed and insect killers)

- Various toxins from processed, mass-produced foods, food coloring, flavoring and flavor enhancers, preservatives, and so on

- Radiation from cosmetic laser surgery*

- Heavy/long-term use of various medications

- Smoking

- Drugs

- Chemotherapy

*Radiation from laser treatments and other sources will result in toxin markings in the iris that are similar to intoxification. The reddish-brown layer on the iris will be particularly thick and, in most cases, will reach the cilliary border and cover all other markings.

Intoxification (autotoxification) is generally self-induced and can be treated. Iris markings indicating this state will disappear as a result of significant changes in diet and after the body detoxifies.

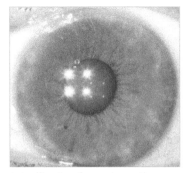

All cases of intoxification will damage "good" intestinal flora; consequently, the "bad" bacteria increase and damage results.

Intoxification from chemotherapy

Light-brown intoxification is congenital and indicates fetal intoxification due to the mother's habits during pregnancy, such as smoking, drugs, bad nutrition, or overuse of medications.

Intoxification markings manifest physically as damage to blood quality, blood toxification, and liver damage. Symptoms can include fatigue, difficulty concentrating, digestive problems due to damaged intestinal flora, anxiety/edginess, headaches, dizziness, nausea, and allergies. Not everyone suffering from these symptoms suffers from intoxification. There are many other causes for these complaints. If intoxification markings appear in the iris and symptoms exist, a connection can be presumed.

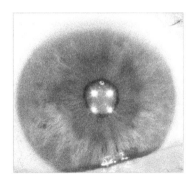

Toxins can always be cleared and the intoxification markings will disappear after detoxifying the body and continuing to lead a healthy lifestyle.

Good bacteria supplements are recommended for the digestive system.

Every toxin-clearing process should include hot baths and perspiration to induce detoxification through the skin.

Consultation with a detoxification expert is recommended.

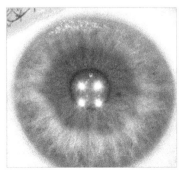

Intoxification

- - - - - -

CHAPTER 7

Central Heterochromia

Central heterochromia indicates a genetic weakness of the liver, pancreas, and spleen and a tendency toward gout and diabetes. It appears as a light orange to reddish ring surrounding the collarette that resembles a ring of small patches joined together.

The ring indicates toxins such as excess sulfur, phosphorous, lead, and mercury. These substances can enter the body as a result of long-term use of dermatological creams in childhood, through foods (sulfur is used to preserve dried fruit), or from environmental toxification.

The central lymphatic ring is located in the same area and indicates the extent of toxification and lymphatic congestion. The lymph cells are overloaded and have difficulty expelling foreign substances from the body. These two rings overlap, and it requires skill to tell them apart.

Congenital heterochromia is genetic; in my experience, it never completely disappears from the eye, even after thoroughly detoxifying the body.

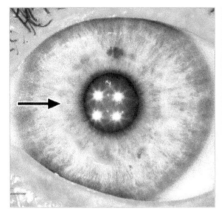
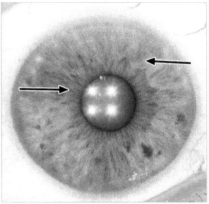

Heterochromia   Detoxification process

CHAPTER 8

Rings on the Iris

Rings crossing the radial structure of the iris can be seen. The color, kind, location, and depth of the rings can indicate the following: sodium ring, lymphatic ring, scurf rim, allergy ring, and anemia ring, each of which are discussed below.

SODIUM RING

The sodium ring is characterized by a white to gray, sometimes bluish, ring surrounding the outer rim of the iris. The sodium ring is dull and is located on the cornea; it appears to be on the edge of the iris but is not part of it. The ring is smeared on the cornea and therefore does not disappear with body detoxing. The sodium ring indicates blood-vessel calcification of the areas indicated by its location. In cases where a sodium ring appears exclusively in the head area (arcus senilis), this indicates calcification of blood vessels specifically in this area.

The thicker and murkier the ring, the more severe the calcification of the blood vessels.

A sodium ring around the iris can indicate the presence or danger of the following:

- Stroke

- Heart failure

- Respiratory damage

- Worsening of existing asthma

- Memory loss

- Hair loss

- Hair whitening

- Sensory and motor disorders in the legs (influenced by calcification of blood vessels in the head)

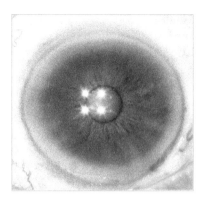

Sodium ring

Take note of the difference between an arcus senilis and a murky gray ring around the head area, which indicates heavy-metal poisoning (such as mercury and lead).

This marking is topostable—indicating local blood-vessel calcification of the area in which the ring appears, as indicated on the iridology chart. A sodium ring generally begins in the head area because many tiny blood vessels are found in this area, and they tend to become blocked first. The next stage is the chest area, followed by the legs. Blood-vessel calcification of the heart and lung area indicates severe asthma.

A sodium ring is created due to disorders in liver functioning and deficient metabolic action of the pancreas.

Blood work of a person with a sodium ring will often show a normal LDL (cholesterol) level. The main indication of a sodium ring is calcification of blood vessels.

Some of the causes of disorders in liver and pancreas functioning and production of cholesterol include the following: 1) consumption of food with high levels of salts and minerals—levels higher than the body is able to process, 2) high self-production of LDL, 3) animal fat and fried food, and 4) emotional causes (see pages 76–77).

In some cases, the client has high cholesterol and triglyceride levels but has no apparent sodium ring in the eye. In these cases, a ring of transparent white jelly will be observed around the iris rim

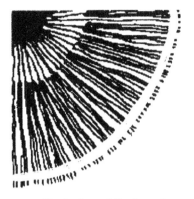

Illustration of Sodium ring

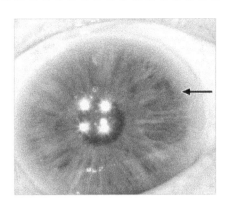

Sodium ring—blood vessel calcification

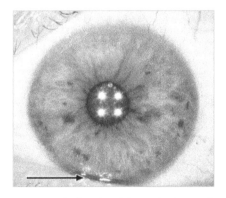

Marking indicating blood cholesterol

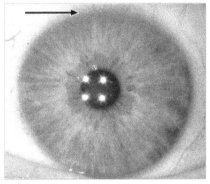

Heavy-metal poisoning

(see illustration). This marking indicates cholesterol/triglycerides in the blood. (A cross-check can be done with information read in the sclera, which shows the current status.)

Generally, a sodium ring appears after age forty. A sodium ring at a younger age indicates the severity of the condition.

Correct treatment of the conditions emphasizes purifying and strengthening the liver and a change in diet: avoid salt and sugar, reduce carbohydrate intake, and reduce fats and trans-fats. Drinking good-quality water is important; low-sodium water is recommended.

A sodium ring will not disappear even after effective treatment.

Note: Sometimes clients will report eating everything, including high sodium and high fat foods, yet they do not have calcified blood vessels or high blood cholesterol. In other cases, clients eat very little sodium and fat or none at all, exercise regularly, and are not over-weight. But in spite of their lifestyle, they have blocked arteries and high cholesterol levels.

The primary physical cause is genetic. People differ in their meta-bolic functioning. Some people tend to produce more cholesterol and blood-vessel calcification than others. In addition, people have congenital differences in their blood vessels. Therefore, a person with wide blood vessels will block up more slowly, leaving sufficient space for blood flow. Others, with narrow blood vessels, can block quickly, even if they follow a healthy diet.

American iridologists claim this to be a precancerous marking.

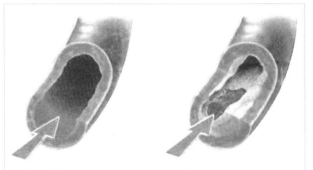

Healthy artery (left): blood flows freely

Calcified artery (right): blood flow impaired

THE EMOTIONAL CAUSE OF BLOOD CHOLESTEROL

After fifteen years of collecting information from thousands of eyes, where I have often seen high cholesterol levels in thin people who exercise regularly and eat healthy diets that limit fatty, fried, and salty food, I have reached an important conclusion: these types have a certain behavioral pattern that creates a "state of accumulation" in their bodies. The common denominator in all these cases is that they are all people who take on a lot of responsibility, act alone, do not let others assist them, and have difficulty delegating. They do not share their feelings and decisions with others.

I questioned these people about their behavior. In every single case, I discovered absolute correlation between the physical phenomena of high cholesterol and the behavior pattern described above. In the same way they accumulate power, control, and unexpressed feelings, cholesterol is accumulated in their blood. Medication is therefore only partially effective. This raises the concept that physical problems cannot be completely resolved without treating the emotional and psychological aspects as well.

LYMPHATIC RING

A lymphatic ring can be white or light to dark brown, depending on the level of lymphatic congestion. The ring can be complete or incomplete and resembles a delicate, dark cloud covering areas of the iris.

The lymphatic ring is located deep inside the iris and therefore disappears when the body is detoxified. The darker and larger the ring, the worse the state of the immune system. The lymphatic system is composed of lymph tracts and lymph nodes. It is first in the line of defense against foreign intruders entering the body; keeping it in good order is therefore imperative.

This ring can appear in every constitution. It is easier to identify in blue eyes because of the contrast between the whitish-brown ring and the blue iris color. In a brown eye, the lymphatic ring will be yellow to gray, depending on the severity of the condition.

Some researchers claim that this marking is topolable and indicates a systemic weakness. Others claim that its location on the iris indicates the specific location of congested lymph nodes, topostable, as follows:

- A lymphatic ring in the upper iris indicates dysfunction of the lymph tracts leading to the head.

- A lymphatic ring in the lower iris indicates dysfunction of the leg lymph nodes.

- A lymphatic ring at the sides of the iris indicates dysfunction of the lymph nodes in the arms, chest, and armpits.

- In women, a particularly dark lymphatic ring in the chest area can indicate the possibility of a malignant breast tumor.

The above argument concerning the location should not confuse the practitioner. The findings should be cross-checked with other markings observed in the eye and with information reported by the client, including laboratory tests. Reach a conclusion after taking all factors into consideration.

After many years of experience, I tend to support the second claim. In my opinion, there is no contradiction between the two claims because the lymphatic ring reflects the state of the immune system, which should be strengthened in both cases.

A lymphatic ring can be observed in two places on the iris:

1. Central Lymphatic ring—parallel to the collarette

2. Peripheral Lymphatic Ring—adjacent to the cilliary border. For example, in a type A2, the ring will be on top of the tophi, and there can be a central lymphatic ring as well, depending on the condition. A lymphatic ring indicates the body's difficulty in ridding itself of toxins and to what extent the immune system has been weakened—according to strength and darkness of its color. In serious cases, it can indicate the development of a malignancy.

Note: Do not base a claim on one single indication. Search for additional markings that support the suspected disorder.

An IC line (immune compromise line) is a significant marking that confirms immune weakness. An IC line is a straight, red line in the sclera that circles a portion of the iris (see illustration below). This line indicates a weak immune system that affects specific systems and organs according to the route the line follows on the sclera chart. (See Chapter 14.)

Note: Lymphatic rings and IC lines fade after correct treatment.

The best way to treat lymphatic disorders is through diet, lymphatic massage, reflexology, herbs, homeopathy, and exercise. If the marking in the eye does not disappear after at least six months of treatment, a serious, long-term disease is indicated.

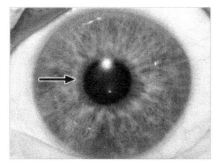 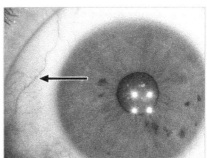

ABOVE LEFT:
Central lymphatic ring

ABOVE RIGHT:
IC line on sclera—weak immune system

RIGHT:
Peripheral lymphatic ring

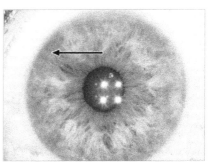

SCURF RIM

The scurf rim is located on the cilliary border and is an inseparable part of it. The rim's color and width provide important information concerning skin functioning and the body's ability to expel toxins through the skin. The skin's functions are as follows:

- Protection
- Sensory organ
- Absorption and secretion

- Respiratory organ
- Controlling body temperature
- Cosmetic

If the scurf rim area is light in color and free of markings, this indicates healthy, properly functioning skin. A person with skin in this condition reacts normally to heat and cold and perspires normally and is therefore well protected from catching a cold and from disease in general.

Malfunctioning skin is indicated by a gray to black ring. A person with skin in this condition does not perspire properly, suffers from lack of fluids, which results in damage to kidney function and increases the probability of kidney stones. In Chinese medicine, the skin is the "third kidney."

Types A2 and A3 have a genetic scurf rim. In some cases, a severe, chronic skin disease develops, and a scurf rim can appear in other constitutions. This is an acquired scurf rim. For example, a scurf rim can develop due to laser hair removal, working near a source of powerful radiation, and working with contaminating chemicals and pesticides.

A very dark, wide scurf rim indicates a precarcinogenic state. I have frequently observed a dark, wide scurf rim in cosmeticians who use chemicals directly on their hands—these substances are absorbed into the body and cause allergies and other damage.

A thick scurf rim in the head area indicates overloading of the brain that can cause the following:

- Lack of concentration
- Difficulty in thinking
- Headaches
- Dandruff
- Tendency to contract head lice

In my experience, a particularly broad scurf rim in a woman's chest area indicates a precarcinogenic state. A particularly thick scurf rim in the foot area indicates severe foot skin problems, such as viral warts, fungi, and eczema.

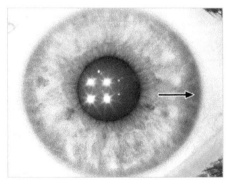

Scurf rim

In psoriasis patients, there may be a congenital scurf rim indicating that the disease is hereditary, or in other cases, no scurf rim at all, but a large number of contraction furrows, indicating that the disease is emotion-based and therefore easier to treat.

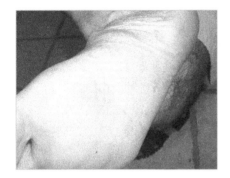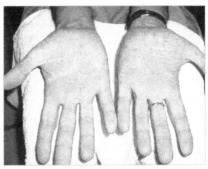

Eczema resulting from a difficult emotional state since childhood.
Acquired scurf rim in the iris.

*"The soul needs spiritual satisfaction
in the same way as the body needs food."*
—FROM THE ZION JERUSALEM CALENDAR

ALLERGY RING

An allergy ring is characterized by a circle of little red consecutive Xs on the sclera, immediately adjacent to the iris. In some cases, a complete ring is formed and, in others, a partial ring. This marking indicates a congenital tendency toward allergies.

A person with congenital allergy tendencies will almost certainly develop symptoms later. Allergies can develop due to overexposure to certain foods, environmental causes, bodily excretions, emotions, and so on. The body overreacts in cases of allergy due to immune-system weakness. In most cases, the process is psychosomatic—an emotional state, trauma, fear, and anxiety create a negative influence on the physical body and trigger the tendency. Therefore, treatment has to address two levels equally: physical and emotional.

The seven principal allergy-causing foods in modern times are as follows (see also Chapter 16):

- Eggs
- Milk
- Peanuts
- Sugars
- Cereals
- Corn
- Soy

Contrary to common knowledge, an allergy can manifest itself in many other forms apart from a cold and a red nose—headaches, frequent colds, pain, irritation, anxiety, impatience, restlessness, lack of concentration, hyperactivity, difficulty making decisions and coping with life, depression, and even severe degenerative diseases.

Treatment with medications and creams repress the symptoms in mild cases but subsequently lead to an outbreak of a more serious disease. Treatment must resolve the root cause of the problem; otherwise clients will return repeatedly, unable to find a long-term solution. If the root cause is not treated, serious diseases will develop later in life. The cause is generally rooted in the client's past or childhood, and treatment should be directed to it.

Unfortunately, Western medicine does not have an all-encompassing solution to allergies. The approach is to distance the person from the source of allergy, which is often impossible (for example, in people who are allergic to the substances their own bodies secrete), or to prescribe medication to suppress the symptoms—an approach that does not properly heal and creates a more serious problem in the future.

Natural medicine, specifically vibrational medicine, has tools that can comprehensively treat the root cause of the allergy and its effect on body and soul. During these treatments, the body learns how to react to the cause of the allergy in a balanced manner and undergoes a kind of corrective experience.

I use a number of vibrational healing methods to treat allergy:

IPEC, EFT, TFT, TAT, and Reconnective Healing, among others, to create a balance of body, mind, and soul.

Identifying an allergy ring at an early age allows us to treat the cause of the allergy before damage is done and to advise the client how to live healthily, thus preventing future difficulties.

> I would like to stress that the advantage of iridology is in its ability to forewarn of future disorders (long before symptoms appear in the body) and thus contribute to improving quality of life.

Note: Iridologists practice complementary medicine; we are not healers. Rather, we assist in balancing body and soul, facilitating the body to achieve a state in which it can heal itself and restore its cells to correct functioning.

Rings on the iris—illustration

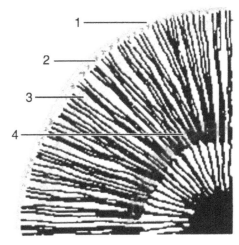

1 Anemia ring   2 Allergy ring   3 Peripheral lymphatic ring   4 Central lymphatic ring

ANEMIA RING

An anemia ring appears as a blue stripe on the sclera, encircling the iris. The width and shade of the ring reflect the severity of the anemia.

Most brown eyes have an anemia ring. These constitutions are haematogenic (blood disorders), and therefore, these types suffer from some degree of anemia.

It requires skill to ascertain if a blue ring circling the iris indicates a degree of anemia that requires attention.

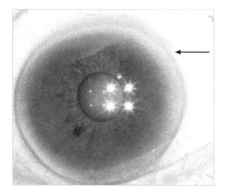
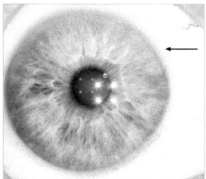

Anemia ring in a brown eye   Anemia ring in a blue eye

CHAPTER 9

The Pupils

The pupil is the black orifice located in the center of the iris, through which light penetrates to the lens and through which we see.

The markings on the iris do not affect our sight with the exception of a pterygium—a fatty membrane that originates on the sclera and grows over the iris, toward the pupil. A pterygium results from overexposure of the eyes to harsh weather conditions: wind, cold, strong sun, and dryness. At some stage, it can obstruct our vision and must be surgically removed. After being removed, a pterygium can regrow.

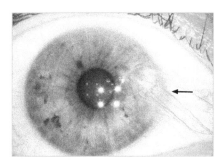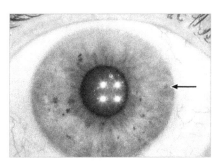

Pterygium before surgery   Pterygium after surgery

Note: When examining the pupils, note their size, color, position, and shape.

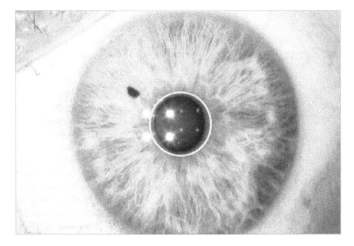

The pupil

Normal pupils are symmetrical. Both pupils should be the same size and color. Pupils in the center of the iris indicate balanced health. They are not too large or too small and are clear, deep, and sharp black.

The pupil responds to light. The pupil's reflex speed indicates the state of the autonomic nervous system. If this reflex is lacking, this indicates damage to the autonomic nervous system. Damage can result from drug use, steroids, or trauma and, in rare cases, can be due to a developing brain tumor.

Note: If the pupil does not react to light, a thorough, conventional medical investigation is imperative.

Changes in the pupil occur due to the following:

- Pupil dilation using special eyedrops for that purpose

- Pathological influences of disease; the perfect circular shape changes and flattened areas and distortions appear, reflecting changes in body functioning

- Medications that contain steroids, psychiatric drugs, narcotics, and the like

- Accidents, traumas, and eye or facial surgery (such as cosmetic nasal surgery)

The pupils also indicate personality traits, as follows:

- **A small pupil** indicates an artistic individual, modest, aesthetic, and loving. An undefined collarette plus a small pupil indicate a humane, sensitive personality; honesty, an artist, an intellectual, a historian, an introvert, or a person who spends a lot of time in thought.

- **A large pupil** plus a symmetrical collarette indicate a person suited to business, someone who wants to "have it all," a mathematician, a person who doesn't spend time in contemplation, acts quickly. Such a person is also restless.

- **A large pupil** indicates a person who is suffering from fatigue or an illness. Occasionally, a large pupil is observed in people suffering from parasites.

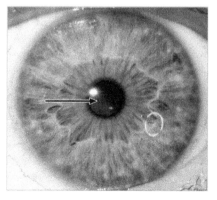

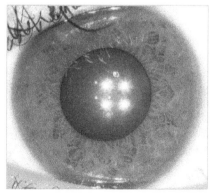

Small pupil   Large pupil

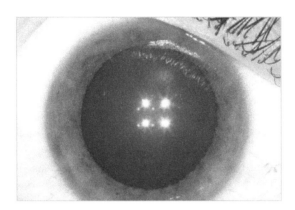

Very large pupil

One large and one small pupil indicate the following possibilities:

- Damage to the nervous system due to long-term use of steroids or drugs

- Hereditary damage to the nervous system, resulting from syphilis in past generations

- Damage resulting from diphtheria

Two well-known eye diseases that can be seen in the aperture of the pupil are cataract and glaucoma. A murky gray pupil indicates cataract. A greenish pupil indicates glaucoma.

During aging, the eye lens becomes cloudy as a result of fat consumption. Western medicine regards cataracts as a natural consequence of aging. Eastern (Chinese) medicine links physiological processes to behavior, nutrition, and the emotional state.

Chinese medicine regards the eye as the twin of the liver. Therefore, all liver functions resulting from nutrition and/or expression or repression of emotions (especially anger) will cause changes in the eye and the pupil. This explains why a cataract can return after being surgically removed, if significant dietary changes are not made. To prevent this, do not consume animal fats, fried food, or oil.

CATARACT

There are two types of cataract:

● **Congenital cataract**—Appears at birth

● **Acquired (developed) cataract**—The most common cause is aging, but other causes are nutritional disorders, X-rays, heat from various sources of radiation (cellular phones perhaps), trauma due to a systemic disease such as diabetes, uveitis, Becker muscular dystrophy, exposure to the sun, or lack of antioxidants.

In both cases, the symptoms of cataracts are:

● Significant, painless deterioration in sight. The level of deterioration depends on where the cloudiness appears on the lens. If the center of the lens becomes cloudy—nuclear cataract—the person will be pleased to discover that reading glasses are no longer necessary.

● Change in diopter of distance and reading glasses

● Bright lighting required for reading

● Deterioration of night vision

● Dazzling by car lights at night

These can be symptoms of other eye disorders as well.

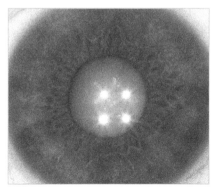

Pupil with cataract—
left eye before surgery

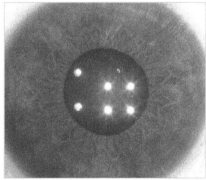

Pupil after cataract surgery—
right eye

GLAUCOMA

Glaucoma is a disease accompanied by increased intraocular pressure and a gradual reduction of the field of vision. Glaucoma is usually the result of blocked drainage of the interocular fluid. There are two types of glaucoma: primary glaucoma (of which there are two subtypes) and secondary glaucoma.

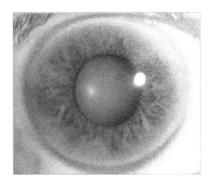

Glaucoma

- **Primary Glaucoma**

  o Acute narrow-angle glaucoma —A sudden, painful rise in intraocular pressure and blurred vision

  o Chronic glaucoma—A gradual rise in intraocular pressure and a gradual loss of vision

- **Secondary Glaucoma** may develop when some other eye disease damages the intraocular fluid flow and causes a rise in intraocular pressure.

Treatment for both types of glaucoma aims at reducing the intraocular pressure. This can be done using eyedrops administered at regular intervals or surgically.

Glaucoma becomes more common with age and is one of the major causes of blindness.

"People who expect to correct nutritional lack by taking supplements, without changing their lifestyle, are like people desiring to be close to God without mending their ways."

—AVI YAACOBOVITZ, HERBALIST

CHANGES IN PUPIL SHAPE

The pupil can change shape in two ways: a round pupil can become oval and/or flattened. Definition of the positioning of the oval/flattened section in relation to the nose/ear is as follows:

A pupil facing:

- The ear—temporal
- The nose—nasal

- The head—cranial
- The legs—caudal

An Oval Pupil

When the pupil is oval (see illustrations on page 92), consider the following options:

1. Vertically axised oval—past stroke or a probable stroke. In my clinical experience, I have seen a vertical oval pupil in people (mainly women) who underwent nose surgery—cosmetic or otherwise.

2. Horizontally axised oval—indicates psychosis or existing or probable paralysis of the lower limbs. I met a sixty-year-old woman with a horizontally axised oval. She was in a wheelchair and all she wanted to know was if there was any chance of her ever walking again. The damage indicated in the pupil showed damage to the central nervous system and, therefore, her condition was irreversible.

3. Oval axised left and upward (from the observers point of view) —disorder of brain motor system function, danger of stroke

4. Oval axised right and upward—suspected disorders of the cerebellum (Meniere's disease—a disorder of the inner ear causing dizziness)

5–6. The axes of both ovals meet at the cranial or caudal point— tendency to paralysis of lower limbs, lumbar, or sacral spinal problems

See the illustrations below.

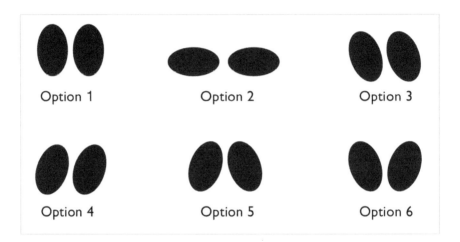

Option 1   Option 2   Option 3

Option 4   Option 5   Option 6

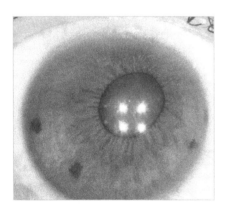

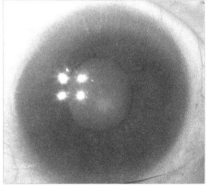

An oval pupil pointing toward   An oval pupil
the nose and upward

"Where there is knowledge there is light."

—LEE CARROL

FLATTENING OF THE PUPIL

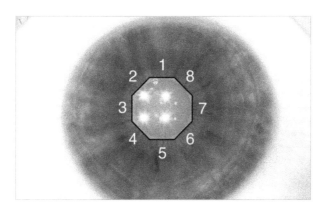

Flattening of the pupil

Flattening of Area 1

- Depression/surrendering to emotional suffering
- Loss of communication due to disorder of the central nervous system
- Hormonal balance disorder
- Electrolyte disorder

Flattening of Area 2

- Inner-ear disorder, particularly of the middle ear (Take brain function into account in this case.)
- Disorder of cervical vertebrae

Note: When the three upper areas of the pupil are flattened, consider brain pathology.

Flattening of Area 3

- Vascular and cardiac disorders
- Lung diseases

Flattening of Area 4

- Liver, gall bladder
- Duodenum
- Rectal and vaginal disorders
- Muscular atrophy
- Osteoporosis of upper limbs

Flattening of Area 5

- Spinal and lower limb disorders
- Urinary system
- Urogenital region

Flattening of Area 6

- Lumber and sacral region
- Genitals

Flattening of Area 7

- Respiratory disorders
- Esophagus
- Trachea
- Bronchi
- Thyroid gland
- Thoracic vertebrae

Flattening of Area 8

- Visual disorders
- Sinus
- Nasal disorders
- Cervical vertebrae

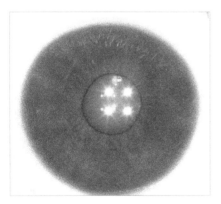 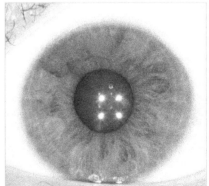

Flattening of the pupil

THE RIM OF THE PUPIL
AND THE INNER PUPILLARY BORDER

The rim of the pupil surrounds the pupilliary border on its inner and outer edge. The markings in this area are continuous. They circle the pupil and for this reason are called "rings."

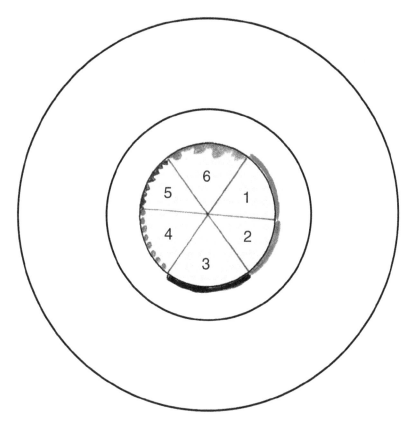

1 Asthenia ring   **2** Absorption ring   **3** Shadow ring
4 Hormonal ring   **5** Neurasthenia ring   **6** Diabetes ring

*"A good meal should include one third food,
one third liquids and one third love."*

—AVI YAACOBOVITZ, HERBALIST

ASTHENIA RING (WEAKNESS)

Positioned on the outer border of the pupil—a delicate ring, ranging from shiny yellow-red to red-brown. This ring indicates a sensitive, gentle person with a tendency to physical and spiritual weakness. The asthenia ring is more common in A5 constitutions but can be found in other constitutions as well, such as A2 and A3.

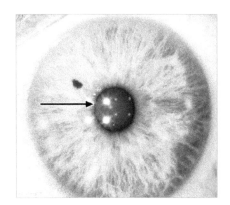 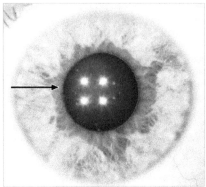

Asthenia ring

"If a man desires to touch God but can't find him, let him warmly hug his mother as she is God's representative on this earth in her devotion, love and transcendence."

—AVI YAACOBOVITZ, HERBALIST

ABSORPTION RING

This brown ring is on the outer border of the pupil. It indicates problems in absorbing vital substances from food into the digestive system.

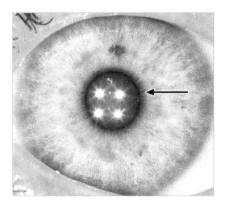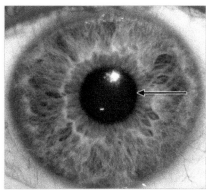

Absorption ring

SHADOW RING

This dark gray to black ring is on the outer border of the pupil. It indicates a family history of cancer—a large number of carcinogenic disorders in the family. In addition, this ring indicates sensitivity to selenium, zinc, and germanium; lack of minerals; and a tendency toward anemia.

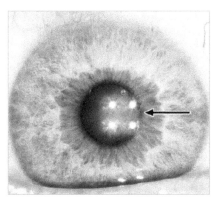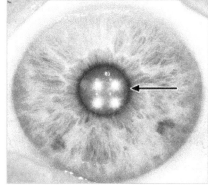

Shadow ring

HORMONE RING (GLANDS)

This ring is on the inner border of the pupil. It is composed of small brown gold beads arranged like a "pearl" necklace. These "pearls" indicate the condition of the hormonal system. In a healthy system, the "necklace" is perfectly spaced, consecutive, and complete. Missing "pearls" in the necklace indicate hormonal disorder.

In my experience, it is important to note the areas where the "pearls" are concentrated around the circumference. Missing parts of the ring indicate hormonal weakness. A missing hormone ring in the fertility area indicates fertility problems in men/women, menstrual disorders/amenorrhea, and menopausal problems. In addition, it indicates premature aging.

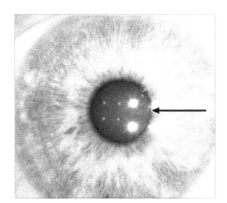
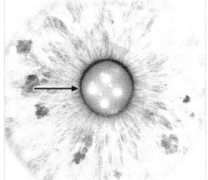

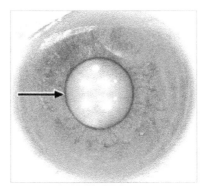

Hormone ring

NEUROSTHENIA RING

This ring resembles flakelike markings facing into the pupil. It indicates a person with weak nerves, consciously unpleasant, who bears grudges and tends to be hysterical.

DIABETES RING

This ring resembles unevenly structured bubbles of "burnt sugar" flowing into the pupil. This is an uncommon marking and indicates a tendency to diabetes. Occasionally, the "bubbles" overlap; this indicates an angry, restless, and unpredictable person.

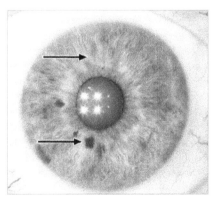

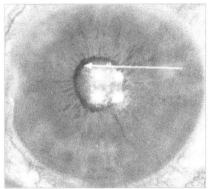

Other markings indicating a tendency   Tendency to diabetes
to diabetes (pigments)

"A crust eaten in peace is better than a banquet
partaken in anxiety."
—AESOP

SERRATED PUPIL

A serrated pupil indicates parasites and worm nests that cause the pupil's shape to change. This indicates irreversible damage to the central nervous system and to the digestive system.

Most parasites enter the body through consumption of beef and pork. Another source is dogs that eat raw meat, develop worms, and pass them on to humans.

Several years ago, I treated an Israeli agronomist who had returned after a long period in Africa. He complained of extreme fatigue and weakness that made it hard for him to stand and forced him to spend most of his time in bed. I observed eye markings indicating parasites and asked him if he had eaten meat that was improperly cooked or stored, or unfamiliar types of meat. He confirmed that he had eaten crocodile meat and recalled that his symptoms had appeared soon after.

There are many types of parasites and worms, some of them microscopic and some of them extremely long—up to several meters in length. They cause damage to the digestive system, to the brain, and to the lungs. Another indication of parasites is radii solaris in the iris (see Chapter 11). In this case, the radii appear almost symmetrically around the iris. This marking also indicates great fatigue and systemic weakness.

Note: White dots on the iris indicate lack of vitamin A.

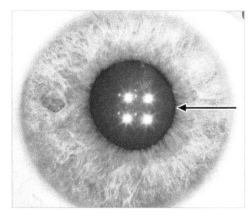

Serrated pupil—parasites

POSITIONING OF THE PUPILS

A physically and emotionally balanced person's pupils are in the center of the iris. It is very common to observe other conditions as follows:

- **Pupil with an upward tendency**—indicates disorders in head functioning

- **Pupil with a downward tendency**—indicates disorders of the kidneys, genitals, legs, and tendency toward hemorrhoids

- **Pupil with a nasal tendency**—indicates a sensitive digestive system, emotional disorders, and difficulty coping with difficult life situations due to communication problems

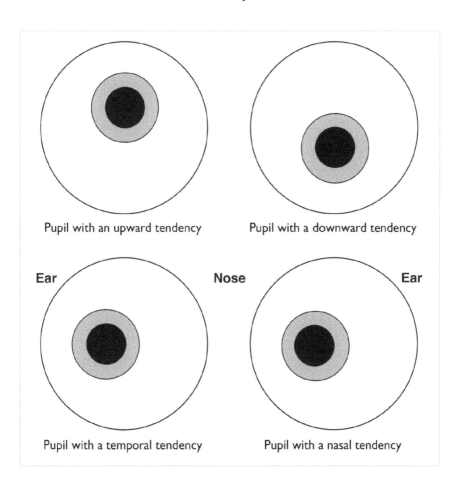

Pupil with an upward tendency | Pupil with a downward tendency

Pupil with a temporal tendency | Pupil with a nasal tendency

- **Pupil with a temporal tendency**—indicates cardiac/respiratory disorders

CHAPTER 10

Pigments

Pigments are "stains" or a group of dots appearing on the iris. Pigments indicate that the body is susceptible to disease, due to accumulated physical and emotional toxins in various organs.

- **Physically**—One can observe the formation and development of pigments over several years, paralleling the resulting health deterioration. Pigments indicate organ weakness due to accumulated toxins (resulting from faulty metabolism, medication, narcotics, chemicals ingested with food, and so on), or a congenital or acquired disorder. Pigments also indicate past illnesses.

- **Emotionally**—Pigments indicate repressed thoughts and emotions.

Many of the pigments on the iris indicate organic weakness and a high probability of future disease.

If there is only a single pigment on the iris, its position on the iridology chart should be noted. This information, combined with information gleaned from interpreting its color, enables us to evaluate where the damage is. However, it does not reveal when disease is going to erupt.

- The more pigments in the eye, the more severe the condition.

- The darker the pigment, the greater the possibility of developing a serious disease.

- If there are more pigments in one eye than the other, do regular checkups, because of the possibility that the organs on one side of the body are significantly weaker than on the other.

- One or more pigments in the stomach or intestinal area, of any color, indicate the possibility of cancer, but with no indication where or when it may occur.

- A pigment adjacent to lacunae indicates an even greater organ weakness than if there is only one visible marking.

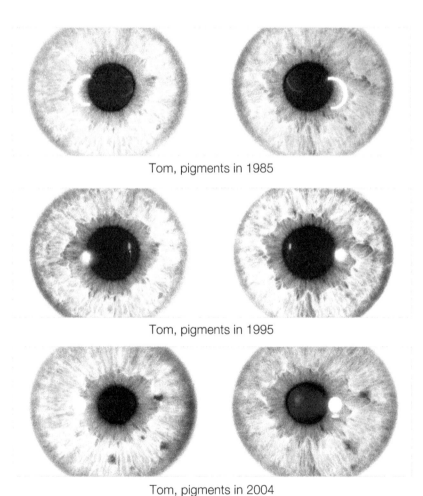

Tom, pigments in 1985

Tom, pigments in 1995

Tom, pigments in 2004

(These pictures are used with the courtesy of Dr. Mehlmauer.)

A suitable detoxing treatment will gradually make the pigments disappear. Within seven years, the eye can become completely clear of signs of intoxification. However, sometimes, pigments remain. A true challenge!

Pigments can have different colors and each color indicates weakened functioning of different organs.

PIGMENTS—INTERPRETATION OF COLOR

Dark Black—Indicates a malignant process. The pigment's placement does not necessarily indicate the affected organ. A small pigment is more dangerous than a large one because it indicates the start of a new process, even though it is easier to treat because it is less established.

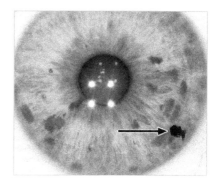

Note: Black pigment is very rare.

Black pigment

Dark Brown—Indicates pancreatic weakness, reduced digestive enzyme production, and difficulty metabolizing carbohydrates. This can result in IGT (borderline diabetes). Small, dark-brown dots, resembling paprika, and covering part of or the entire iris indicate active diabetes.

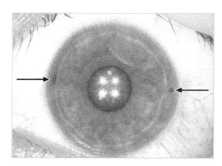

Brown pigment in a brown eye

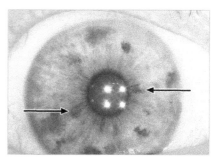

Pigment in the stomach area

Reddish-Brown—Indicates pancreatic weakness combined with gall bladder weakness. This indicates a tendency to produce gallstones or benign tumors in the gall bladder. These can slow the flow of gall fluids and/or produce a tendency toward stenosis and narrowing of the gall ducts.

Reddish-Brown to Orange—Indicates liver disorders and malfunctioning and difficulty in excreting toxins entering the body from a diet loaded with chemicals and fat.

Orangey-Yellow—The spleen is weakened due to overloading through consumption of animal fat and rapid eating. There can also be immune disorders that cause long-term infections and exhaust the spleen.

Straw Yellow—A dull yellow that indicates kidney function disorders due to inflammation and difficulty excreting toxins.

Strong Yellow to Gold—This pigment in the head area of the iris, above the intestine, indicates a tendency toward diabetes.

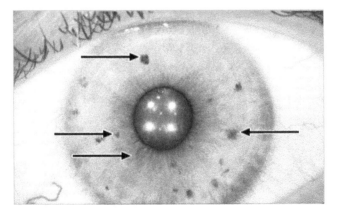

A variety of pigments

Note: A yellow aura in the head area indicates learning disabilities.

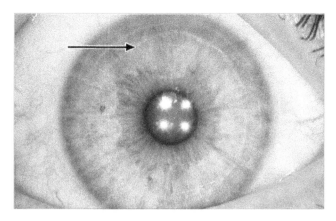

Learning disabilities

Treating people with pigments in their eyes

- Eat plenty of organic fruit and vegetables. A high percentage of raw food is recommended.

- Avoid milk and other dairy products, particularly high-fat cheeses.

- Avoid foods containing preservatives, food coloring, and other chemicals; avoid alcohol, cigarettes, narcotics, and the like.

- Drink plenty of good-quality filtered water.

- Use detoxifying herbs.

- Spend time in nature; take alternate hot and cold baths.

- Visit the beach frequently; relax by dipping your feet in the water.

- Spiritual work, developing awareness and clearing negative emotions from the past influences the future.

I check the location of prominent pigments and single lacunae (or both) in the three most important areas:

- The heart area - The pancreatic area - The liver area

Suspicious markings in these areas require immediate attention, before dealing with anything else.

CHAPTER 11

● ● ● ● ● ●

Radii Solaris

A radii solaris is a dark line originating from the pupil or the collarette, continuing along the stroma, and terminating at the cilliary border. These lines indicate toxins in an organ located somewhere along the line (according to the iridology chart).

The origin of the line indicates the problem's source. Its termination (pointing toward the iris rim) indicates the organ affected by the problem—for example:

- A radii solaris originating from the stomach and leading to the head indicates headaches caused by digestion.

- A radii solaris originating from the collarette and leading to the head indicates headaches caused by pressure on the cervical nerves due to stress.

An iridology analysis always fascinates me. One glance can suffice to locate the source of headaches that may have caused years of suffering and intensive use of painkillers (which damage the liver). Locating the root of the problem enables us to treat the source and not just the symptoms, as is common in conservative methods.

Radii solaris all over the iris indicate worms. In Chinese medicine, there is a connection between the intestine and the respiratory system and, therefore, respiratory disorders (such as asthma) and significant fatigue will also be present.

Note: Worms in children can cause hyperactivity.

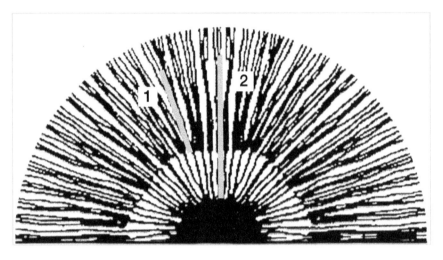

1 Radii solaris originating from the collarette
2 Radii solaris originating from the stomach

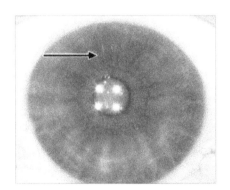
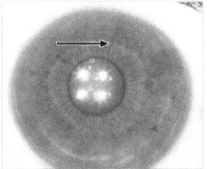

Radii solaris originating from   Radii solaris originating from
the collarette   the stomach

"If a man wants to live a true life he should see himself
as having been resurrected for a few years."
—AVI YAACOBOVITZ, HERBALIST

* * * * * *

CHAPTER 12

Contraction Furrows

Contraction furrows are shaped like "hoops" crossing the stroma and are found between the collarette and the cilliary border. In most cases, the hoops are divided into sections.

Contraction furrows are formed by contraction of the stroma as a result of pressure from the nervous system. This pressure can be caused by great stress or a reaction to a traumatic event that leaves its mark in the physical and emotional bodies.

A trauma is the result of intense fear, sudden or ongoing stress, and the body's reaction to various forms of violence, surgery, accidents, emotional or physical abuse, loss, serious disease, and more.

In some cases, these contractions create a complete hoop that circles the entire iris. A "complete hoop"—a complete contraction—can be found in business people or students who are under long-term stress.

The path of the furrow indicates the organ or system affected by the cause of the contraction. For example, a contraction furrow passing through the brain area indicates pressure in the head, headache, or any other symptom relating to the head, as a result of the trauma.

Most people have more than one contraction furrow in their iris. (We can presume that most people experience more than one trauma in life.) This does not mean that people without contraction furrows have not experienced traumas. However, those who do have the furrows have definitely experienced trauma at some time.

CONTRACTION FURROWS IN THE EYE
AS INDICATORS OF TRAUMA

After years of analyzing thousands of eyes, I believe that contraction furrows reflect the exact time frame that traumatic events occurred during a person's life. This information enables us to focus treatment on emotional issues and points us directly to the events that caused the disorders. Traumatic events leave their mark on a person's psyche and can result in a serious physical disease, behavioral problems, and emotional blockages, which even after many years still affect everyday functioning.

Years of research have taught me that traumas are recorded in the eye in chronological order. The first traumas are marked by contraction furrows adjacent to the cilliary border. As the person ages, traumas are recorded closer to the collarette. Based on this understanding, I have constructed a "time axis," starting from the cilliary border and ending at the collarette. The length of the axis equals the person's age.

The year a trauma occurred is the point at which the contraction furrow crosses the time axis. Each of these cross points indicates a trauma. The axis can be moved all around the iris and will map the organs affected by traumatic events. The results are precise.

My clients have reported amazing accuracy in pinpointing the year of the traumatic event. Client responses are often dramatic. The confirmation of the discovery, the amazement, and the uncontrolled tears resulting from revealing events that the client herself or himself may have repressed for years and might not even remember until I bring up the subject touches the clients deeply. The ability to pinpoint the exact year of the trauma spares the client unnecessary searching and suffering, and saves time.

In many cases, the client cannot remember the event—people tend to repress painful events, particularly if the psyche is unable to cope with the pain. The advantage of my system is its accuracy and ease, and that it enables the practitioner to direct the treatment to specific events without wasting precious time.

A focused emotional clearing is made possible by saving much time and obtaining fast, positive results. Emotional clearing practitioners could benefit greatly from this tool.

Some examples of my clients with a contraction furrow include:

- I.A. has a contraction furrow at age twelve—she had been sexually abused, but had never told a soul. The experience impaired her ability to have relationships with men.

- P.Y. has a contraction furrow at age thirty-two—she had had a traumatic birth experience, giving birth to a child with severe congenital defects. Up until our session, she was not aware of how deeply this had affected other aspects of her life.

- M.G. has a contraction furrow at age thirteen—the age at which he immigrated to Israel and experienced trauma adapting to a new language and society.

These and other events, such as marriage, divorce, death, and long-term physical abuse, result in contraction furrows appearing all over the iris, crossing most of the organs and affecting the person for many years.

Another aspect I am researching at this time is that the same time axis can supply information concerning the nine fetal months.

Note: *The above information is the result of many years of research. Please respect the work invested and treat it with integrity. Do not use this material and information without first receiving guidance and permission, in writing, from myself, Dr. Miriam Garber, Ph.D., MBMD.*

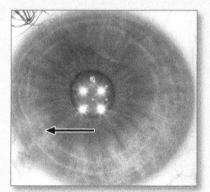 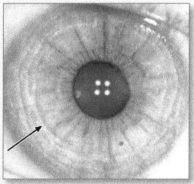

Contraction furrows

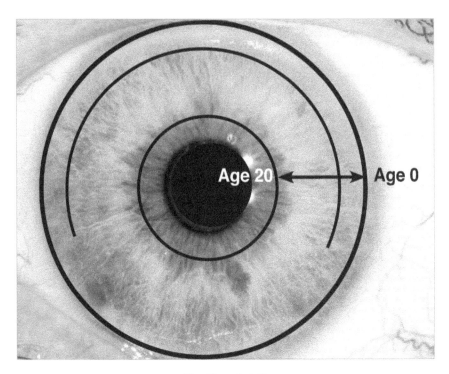

The Time Axis©

If the client is twenty years old, the contraction furrow crosses the time axis at the age of five. We can conclude that a traumatic event that affected the thyroid (see iris chart) occurred at age 5.

*"If a man desires a good marriage, he should aspire that
the equator should not be run between him and his partner
but between the two of them and the whole of creation."*

—AVI YAACOBOVITZ, HERBALIST

CHAPTER 13

— — — — — —

Precancerous Markings

Iridology enables us to glean deep-seated information from the iris, which bears markings that indicate precancerous processes. The markings reflect a process comprised of several factors that together indicate development of neoplastic cells (abnormal cells). Our bodies constantly produce these cells, but a healthy immune system destroys them. Consequently, most of us do not have cancer. However, a person with precancerous signs in their iris has a weak immune system, which is unable to cope with all its tasks for various reasons.

I believe the main reason the immune system is unable to cope lies in the energy field consequently affecting our emotions, which influence our lifestyle, behavior, beliefs, decisions, and actions. The human body is intelligent; it is designed to self-heal if not obstructed by such blocks as fears, limiting belief systems, and negative self-image—all of which can be present from birth or acquired later in life.

"All is foreseen and the freedom of choice is granted."
—THE ETHICS OF THE FATHERS CHAP 3, 15

A CHANGE IN THOUGHT EFFECTS A CHANGE IN DISEASE PATTERNS

People are born with genetic tendencies. When discussing diseases or symptoms with a client, I often hear things like: *My mother also has . . . My father behaves and thinks as I do . . . My grandmother/grandfather also has . . .* and so on. In such cases, I point out that mental patterns, behavioral traits, and beliefs are passed from generation to generation, and in cases where they are negative or limiting, and unchanging, we cannot expect their influence on future generations to be any different. In other words, the same thoughts and the same beliefs will always produce the same results.

A change in thought, belief, and behavior is required to achieve a change in the pattern of disease that passes from generation to generation. For example, people live with half-truths and have difficulty expressing what they truly feel, think, or desire. If a person believes that emotions should not be revealed, and that frustration must not be expressed because that is how it has been in the family for generations, there is a good chance that s/he will live a life of frustration and repressed emotions.

The difference between desire and reality creates frustration, and frustration weakens the immune system. The first effect is the body's reduced ability to withstand "intruders," some of which are always present in a dormant state. These include microscopic parasites (carried in the blood), viruses, bacteria, worms, fungi, and so on, all of which are proven causes of serious illness. Others include:

- Childhood traumas, war traumas, emotional traumas (such as death, divorce, or loss)

- Long-term anger and pain

- Chronic fear and anxiety

- Sexual abuse, physical abuse, long-term emotional abuse

- Genetic patterns

- Environmental pollution

- Various types of radiation: mobile phones, microwaves, antennas, televisions, computers, X-rays, ultrasounds, MRIs, CTs, sunrays, and other types of radiation that "experts" claim are harmless (I disagree)

- Foods saturated with chemicals to increase shelf-life and salability, and to improve taste and visual appeal
- Lack of physical exercise and many other factors

All these produce toxins that obstruct the healthy flow of energy through the body. It sometimes amazes me how the body survives under such a burden.

Emotions and substances are composed of energy frequencies. Energy is composed of particles that affect one another and act in coordination with one another by transmitting information and light through an infinite universal network of energy, which is beyond time and space. This can be proved by observing the influence that past events have on the present. Our cells remember events from the moment of conception (and even before) to the present day. These events are stored in the cellular memory, together with all their negative effects, and are activated under specific circumstances. As a result, intracellular communication is interrupted, inner balance (homeostasis—preservation of inner balance) is disturbed and disease results.

In conclusion: people are responsible for their own diseases. In some cases, the trigger stems from the conscious part of the brain, but in most cases, it stems from the unconscious and the subconscious. If I take it a step further, for those who believe in this concept, the soul's plan and consent on how to live this life and what to learn from it determines the part all the factors listed above will play in helping to manifest the aim of our existence on earth.

All the above-listed motivating factors combine to form the vehicle for manifesting the objectives of the soul that dwells in the physical body. I am aware that it is not easy to accept the idea that we should take responsibility for everything that happens to us. People are used to consulting doctors and expecting medical science to cure them. But the secret of healing lies in our own hands. The responsibility is completely our own. He who is in the chest of life is the only one who can turn the key to the chest from within, open the door, and free himself.

I believe that if we heal our emotions and psyche, the body will be able to heal the physical cells—if it's not too late.

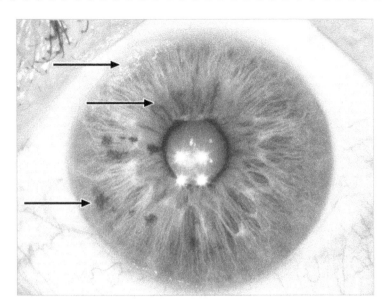

Precancerous signs

Examine the following list of markings to evaluate if the potential for malignant tumors exists. A malignant tumor can develop if all or most of the listed markings appear in the iris and the sclera. This information must be cross-checked with the client's complaints, family history, and social/emotional/psychological/neural circumstances, including self-expression and progress in achieving one's life goals. If the battle to fulfill life's missions is difficult and life does not flow harmoniously, the body will wear out and age earlier.

All of the markings listed below are warning signs of a precancerous condition. The more markings found in the eye and the more negative the client's outlook on life, the greater the chance of becoming ill.

- A particularly dark and wide scurf rim

- A thick cholesterol ring (sodium ring)

- A dark central and peripheral lymphatic ring

- Intoxification

- Significant environmental pollution markings

- Shadow ring

- Black pigment

- Many pigments or particularly dark pigments

- Pigments in the stomach area

- Sclera markings, indicating a weak immune system (IC lines) and additional markings indicating tumors

- Complementary markings in the iris and the sclera; that is, radiation markings, parasite markings, and last but not least, contraction furrows that act as the base and trigger that activate the physical symptoms

- Lacunae steps, neoplasm, torpedo, beait, asparagus

PART THREE

Complementary Information

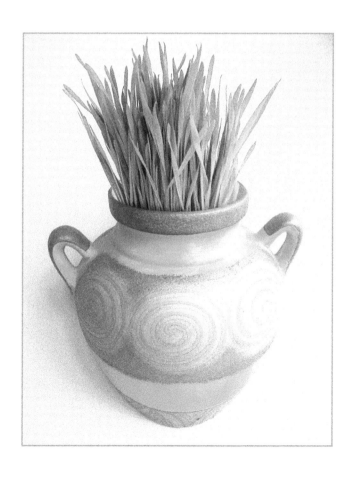

CHAPTER 14

An Introduction to Sclerology

Sclerology is the science of translating the markings on the white of the eye—the sclera—to accurately evaluate the client's health. This practice was developed in China thousands of years ago. In ancient times, the Chinese identified a reflection of the twelve meridians in the sclera. The meridians are channels that carry nourishing energy to all of the bodily systems. Along these meridians are the acupuncture points that are in use today by modern acupuncturists.

The most renowned iridologists in the world today who use sclerology include Leonard Mehlmauer, ND, from San Diego, California (whom I studied with in the United States) and Jack Tipps, ND, from Austin, Texas. I first studied this system in Israel in 1993 with Dr. Shlomo Schlezinger.

THE MARKINGS

The markings consist of red and blue lines, brown dots and marks, and other patches of red, black, blue, white, gray, and yellow. These markings indicate both physiological and emotional states. When a healing process begins in an organ or bodily system, healing signs can immediately be observed in the sclera.

Every sign indicates a pathology developing in the body in real time. Sclera markings appear very quickly, almost immediately, but never completely disappear—even if the physical pathology has healed completely. When the healing process is complete, the specific sclera markings diminish in caliber and brightness (with adequate purification procedures). The sclera markings remain as historical markers.

The appearance of sclera markings indicates a process that is happening right then.

IRIDOLOGY AND SCLEROLOGY

Iridology indicates genetic tendencies and chronic processes. The information from the sclera completes the picture of the present state and helps us understand more accurately which genetic tendencies remain dormant and which have become active. Another advantage of sclerology is that it enables us to see from where a specific pathology stems, what its source organ is, which organs are affected along the way, and which is the ultimate organ or system suffering from the process.

Sclerology, combined with iridology and verification of the findings by blood tests or other means such as urine testing or X-ray, enables us to give a broad, in-depth, and reliable diagnosis of the source of physical and emotional disorders. It must not be forgotten that, in many cases, sclera markings will appear long *before* lab tests can identify the problem. This is because the body's reactions to internal and external changes are extremely subtle. Lab tests identify a pathology when it is at an advanced stage and, in many cases, only when the disease has manifested in the physical body.

As in iridology, a sclerology chart shows all of the organs and bodily systems for identification. Combining knowledge of the markings in both iris and sclera gives the iridologist a powerful tool: the ability to discover the source of a client's suffering without the use of invasive means. I teach both iridology and sclerology at my School of Natural Healing.

Sclera Markings

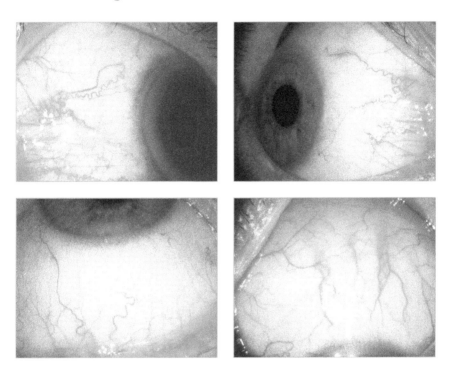

Sclera

CHAPTER 15

Techniques of Eye Examinations

There are two aspects to the technique of eye examinations:

1. Professional etiquette

2. The examination tools

PROFESSIONAL ETIQUETTE

The examination process is an intimate interaction between practitioner and client. Treat the client with respect and politeness. The practitioner must observe the following basic rules:

- Maintain personal hygiene

- Keep clean surroundings

- Seat oneself opposite the client in a respectable manner—distance, body posture, and leg placement

- Behave and speak with modesty

- Offer a detailed explanation of the upcoming examination process

- Take into consideration that the examination process can cause the client discomfort; offer optional intervals for resting

- Adapt the examination process to the client's needs (for example, people with disabilities, those who are religiously observant, and children)

- Explain all stages of the examination process to the client, including the possibility of taking a break to let the eye recover from being illuminated

THE EXAMINATION TOOLS

Magnifying Glass and Flashlight

- The flashlight should be held in one hand, at the side of the client's face.

- Illuminate the iris only from the side to avoid damaging the eye.

- Hold the magnifying glass in the other hand and gradually bring it closer to the eye until you can see the eye clearly.

- Maintain the same order for the right/left eye.

Magnifying Glass with a Built-in Flashlight

Bring the magnifying glass closer to the client's eye, making sure not to dazzle the client.

CHAPTER 16

— — — — — —

Foods That Cause Allergies and Sensitivity

*"Our food should be our medicine
and our medicine should be our food."*
—HIPPOCRATES, THE FATHER OF MEDICINE

Many symptoms of illness like headache, abdominal pain, skin rashes, tiredness, etc., are attributed by the western medicine to certain diseases, which might be right. However, these symptoms can also be present as a result of an allergy to foods, food additives, medications, environmental factors like seasons, all kinds of natural and artificial substances, and reactions to various emotions, fears, and traumas. They can even be caused by an allergy to substances naturally produced by the body, including neurotransmitters, hormones, body fluids, and physiological processes.

The main problem with food allergy is that people cannot avoid certain foods for a lifetime, and the problem with body substances or processes is that there is no way to escape them. Therefore, there is a need for creative methods in order to heal the person.

During my long practice of allergy treatments, most of the symptoms disappeared as a result of allergy neutralizing modalities like IPEC (Integrated Physical and Emotional Clearing), EFT, TAT, and PEAT (Primordial Energy Activation and Transcendence) and other methods.

The following foods are not recommended for types A1, A2, and A3:

- Alcohol
- Bananas
- Beans, chickpeas
- Bicarbonate of soda
- Black tea
- Carbonated drinks
- Cheese (except goat-milk cheese)
- Chemical taste and aroma enhancers
- Citrus fruit (except lemons)
- Corn oil
- Eggplant, tomatoes (except very ripe ones), green peppers, potatoes
- Flour (whole wheat, white)
- Food coloring
- Lima beans
- Meats (except a limited amount of chicken and turkey)
- Melon and mangos
- Pistachio and cashew nuts
- Preservatives
- Salted fish, sole, caviar, salmon, and crab
- Semolina, wheat bran, seven-grain mix
- Sesame seed oil
- Tomato juice, ketchup
- Vinegar, vegetables pickled in vinegar or brine

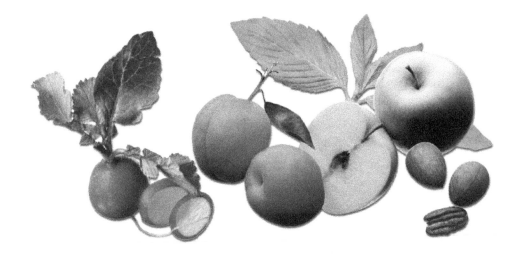

CHAPTER 17

Case Studies—
Images and Discussions

This eye belongs to a male in his mid-forties who is considerably overweight and suffering from high blood pressure. He is not particularly nutrition-literate and functions at a high level of emotional stress for most of the day. His face is flushed, and he suffers from fatigue. He has respiratory difficulties and has deliberated for many years on what he should do with his life.

Markings observed in the eye: Connective tissue weakness, lower back weakness, weak immune system. High level of uric acid in the blood, joint pain, weak thyroid gland.

Signs of intoxification: Signs in stomach area, as a result of taking medication, resulting in a severe lack of digestive enzymes. Lacunae observed in the heart and respiratory area.

Diabetes: Notice the gold pigments in the head area. Markings indicating sinusitis. Weakness of lungs and markings indicating past infections. Arcus senilis—sodium ring in the head area. Lymphatic congestion—notice peripheral lymphatic ring surrounding the iris.

Liver weakness: Notice pigments and transverse fibers. This person is bothered by repetitive thoughts, has a tendency toward anemia, and has difficulty initiating changes in his life.

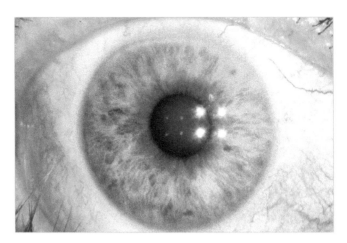

Right eye, A3 + A4

CASE STUDY NO. 2

This eye belongs to a fifty-eight-year-old man suffering from migraines, pain in the bones, and hypochondria. His pupil has a leftward tendency, indicating digestive problems, and an absorption ring can also be observed. He has lacunae in the stomach area and widening of the intestine. This indicates slow intestinal function, precancerous symptoms (dark scurf rim), and sensitivity of the lower-back vertebrae.

A dark pigment in the stomach area (precancerous signs) indicates the possibility of a malignant growth (when and where the disease may appear is unknown). Liver and pancreas weakness can also be observed.

The headaches are caused by contraction of muscles in the neck area (see radii solaris in the head area). Contraction furrows indicate long-term emotional stress and past traumatic periods that still affect the head area.

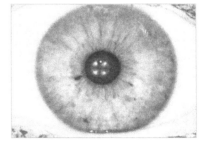

Left eye A2 + A3 + A4

CASE STUDY NO. 3

This eye belongs to a forty-two-year-old woman. She complained of severe digestive problems, severe emotional stress, difficulty falling asleep, and irritability.

Particularly prominent markings in her eye indicate a tendency toward fear and anxiety, as well as a tendency toward headaches and hormonal disturbances.

A large, slightly flattened pupil with flattening at 9, 4, and 5 o'clock indicates thyroid weakness, extreme fatigue, weakness of the small intestine and the sigmoid, and liver weakness (see the color green visible under the brown).

Five to six contraction furrows indicate extremely severe emotional stress, with a tendency toward nervous breakdowns. This stress has been a constant in her life and still continues.

Several of the complementary medical methods I use can help her. Recommended treatments:

- Homeopathy
- Healing herbs
- IPEC—neutralization of allergy and sensitivities, emotional balancing
- Reconnective Healing

- Bio-orgonomy
- Reflexology
- Bach Flower Remedies
- Personal awareness
- Diet change, including macrobiotic foods

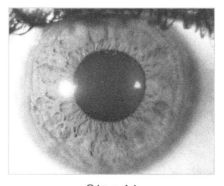

C1a + A4

CASE STUDY NO. 4

This eye belongs to a seventy-year-old woman. The very small pupil indicates a highly stressed and introverted person.

She has significant intoxification—fatigue, lack of concentration, memory difficulties (see sodium ring in the head area as well).

Lighter areas indicate mineral shortage. There is severe pancreatic and liver weakness (see open lacunae originating in the intestinal area), high blood pressure, cholesterol, and hardening of blood vessels all over the body, specifically in the head area.

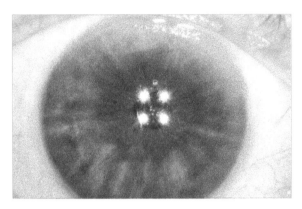

Right eye B2 + A4

CASE STUDY NO. 5

This eye belongs to a farmer in his late sixties or early seventies. He had sprayed his fields with pesticides for many years and breathed in the fumes. He is overweight and suffers from fatigue and aching joints. He drags one leg.

He was severely traumatized at sixteen years old when his brother was injured in war. That was the first time he experienced feeling helpless in the face of tragedy. He was traumatized again at age twenty when he was discharged from the army. He felt unable to face having to transfer from a military to a civilian framework and the need to support himself financially. He is a very shy and sensitive person and tends to take everything to heart.

Intoxification caused by the pesticides can be observed. The color of the iris has changed from blue to gray as a result of years of inhaling pesticides. The large amount of pigments indicates liver weakness, while the pigment in the stomach area indicates a tendency toward cancer. His brother and sister died of cancer, and there is a family history of the disease. Lacunae and white fibers indicate an acidic body and phlegm.

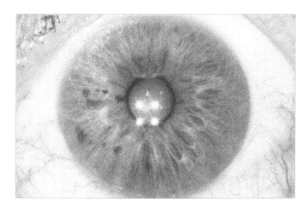

A4

Photos from Additional Case Studies

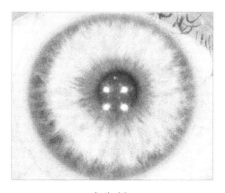

Arthritis

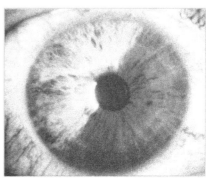

Split constitutions

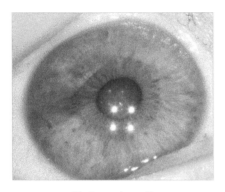

Flattened pupil

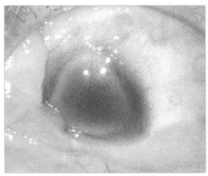

Congenital defect

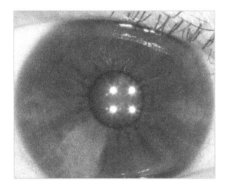

Lack of minerals and congenital
emotional weakness

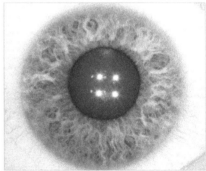

Congenital emotional weakness

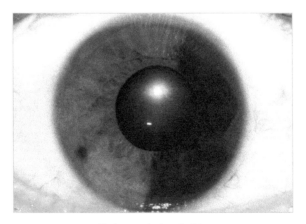

Color variation in iris

Conclusion

This book has presented you with the basics of iridology. As you have seen, the markings in the iris accurately reflect many different conditions. Experience and skill are required to translate the observed markings into practical knowledge. If you are new to iridology, your work is just beginning. This book opens the door to a wonderful world. Take advantage by exploring its paths and harvesting its fruits.

If you are a practitioner who is already using this fascinating method, I am certain that you have found helpful information throughout these pages to clarify and enhance your knowledge. I hope that you have also thought of ways to solve the health problems presented here.

People who come to have their eyes analyzed have a wide range of symptoms that do not always seem related. Using the definition of constitutions, iridology offers an explanation. I hope this book will inspire medical practitioners everywhere to start using this tool to provide satisfactory answers to people who would like to know the source of their ailments. I have no doubt that it is just a matter of time before the medical institutions recognize the value of iridology and then . . . "the sky's the limit."

Iridologists from all over the world meet for mutual enrichment and information exchange. These meetings have made it possible for me to present you with this wealth of information. I hope you have enjoyed reading this book as much as I enjoyed researching and writing it and that you will put the information to good use.

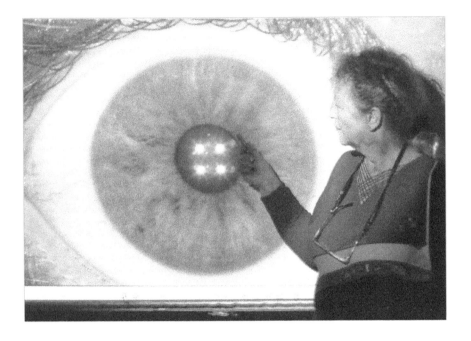

Foundations of an Ideal Life According to the Holistic Approach of Neil Graham*

Life in nature: Spending time in fresh air with plenty of negative ions. Filling the lungs with oxygen. Restricted exposure to sunlight.

Peace of mind: Have a rewarding occupation. Cultivating hobbies, developing a sense of humor, and making time for recreation.

Human relations: Sharing life with loved ones, leading an active social life, cultivating friendships, fellowship and benevolence with others . . . a feeling of belonging.

Natural nutrition: Matched to the client's individual needs, including vitamins, minerals, enzymes, amino acids, and healing herbs.

Draining waste: Through the skin, lungs, kidneys, and digestive system. Internal and external healing cleansing processes such as colonics.

General ecology: Environmentally friendly, no pollution of air, food, and water. Clean and comfortable living conditions, avoiding radiation, toxins, chemical medications, and allergens.

---

* Adapted by Miriam Garber, Ph.D., MBMD

Bio-rhythm: coordinating lifestyle with nature's rhythm: climate, seasons, day and night, sufficient rest and sleep at the right time of day.

Skeletal symmetry: regular physical activity suited to the individual's needs. Correct use of the body in everyday life.

The Twelve Bodily Systems and Their Functions

The Skeletal System

All bones, cartilage and joints

Support and protect the body, enable limbs to swing, store minerals, produce red blood cells

The Muscular System

All the body's muscle tissue

Aid body movement, produce heat, maintain body alignment

The Respiratory System

Lungs, trachea, bronchial tubes, and alveoli

Supply oxygen, exhale carbon dioxide, control and balance alkaline/acid level

The Skin System

Skin, hair, nails, fat, and sweat glands

Body temperature control (heat/cold), waste excretion, pressure, react to pain and touch

The Lymphatic System

Spleen, thymus gland, appendix, tonsils, lymph nodes, and lymph ducts

Filter blood, produce white blood cells, increase immunity to disease, return protein to cardiovascular system

The Reproductive System

Testes, ovaries, semen, ovum, and breasts

Reproduction of the organism

The Circulatory System

Heart, blood, and blood vessels

Transport oxygen and nutrients to cells, transport waste and CO_2 from the cells, balance acidity/alkalinity

The Defecation System

The large intestine

Final absorption of nutrients and fluids, produces certain vitamins, produces and excretes feces

The Glandular System

Pineal gland, hypothalamus, hypophysis, thyroid and parathyroid, thymus, adrenal glands, pancreas, ovaries, and testes

Control bodily functions by transporting hormones through blood vessels and the nervous system

The Digestive System

Mouth, esophagus, stomach, duodenum, small intestine (excluding the large intestine, which is part of the defecation system), salivary glands, liver, gall bladder, and pancreas

Mechanical and chemical (enzymatic) decomposition of food, supply essential nutrients to cells

The Nervous System

Brain, spine, nerves, sensory organs—eyes and ears

Nervous signals controlling bodily functions. Sensory and motorial sensation

The Urinary System

Kidneys, urethra, urinary tract, and bladder

Remove fluid waste from body, control blood chemistry, fluid and electrolyte balance, acidity/ alkaline

Minerals Categorized by Organ Utilization

Every organ needs a specific mineral to enable its proper functioning —for example:

- The stomach needs sodium.
- The intestine needs magnesium.
- The liver needs iron.
- The thyroid gland needs iodine.
- The spleen needs fluoride.
- The pancreas needs zinc.
- The muscles need potassium.

Black patches or "rubbed" areas on the iris indicate the lack of a specific mineral required by a particular organ, according to the iris chart. All the minerals listed below can be supplied through food.

Calcium (Ca). Repairs bone fractures. An essential mineral for bones. Found in sesame, almonds and other nuts, cabbage, carrots, comfrey, bone meal pills, eggshell, and calcium pills. (Eggshell for ingestion is prepared as follows: thoroughly soak washed eggshell overnight in lemon juice or cider vinegar; in the morning, drink the liquid along with the eggshell.)

Fluorine (Fl). Strengthens the spleen. Can be found in unpasteurized milk and pomelo fruit.

Iodine (I). Anti-fear; needed for proper thyroid functioning. Found in sea fish, seaweed, onion, and egg yolk.

Iron (Fe). Needed for liver function. For treating weakness. Found in molasses and floridex, both of which are good for pregnant women. Not all cases of anemia indicate lack of iron. Iron pills are not always recommended as they may cause digestive problems.

Magnesium (Mg). Relaxant. Calms the intestines and nerves. Found in yellow fruit and vegetables, especially yellow figs, corn flour, and yellow squash.

Manganese (Mn). Needed for the brain and the ability to love. Found in almonds and other nuts.

Phosphorus (P). Required for the skin and brain (thought) and for fortifying the skin and brain. Found in proteins, grains, lecithin, and egg yolk.

Potassium (K). For muscles and equilibrium—grace. Found in many fruits and vegetables (especially in bitter vegetables), such as celery, bitter herbs, spinach, watercress, and potato peel soup.

Sodium (Na). For treatment of stomach disorders. Increases vitality and youthfulness. Found in goat's milk, celery, okra, figs, and mutton bone soup (bone broth).

Sulfur (S). People with sensitive skin and people with red hair who anger easily have plenty of this mineral; it is recommended for people with opposite characteristics. It can "ignite" an apathetic person's brain and body. Found in animal protein, vegetables of the cabbage family such as broccoli, cauliflower, and cabbage. Not recommended for people with digestive problems as it can cause flatulence.

Personality Analysis Through Examination

A personality analysis through an examination of the iris and the marks on the white of the eye enables the iridologist to reveal a client's full potential. The ability to see the client's innate abilities and to what extent he or she has realized that potential gives the client a valuable, authentic, and reliable measure of how well he or she has used that potential. This enables the client to reevaluate how he or she wishes to continue in life, with the power to fully use his or her inherent abilities and to expand and extend previous (subjective) limitations.

I invite you to make use of this powerful tool. It will help open your client's mind to who he or she really is and to their previously hidden talents and abilities.

Personality Analysis helps clients:

- Unleash their potential

- Improve relationships

- Discover a personality-suited career

- Select the employee best suited to the job

- Understand in-depth what motivates your daily life

- Understand how your personality controls your behavior

- Discover why you're suffering and how you can be released

- How to step beyond your limitations

- Create a fulfilling career, family, and social life

References

Andrews, John. *Emotional Approaches in Iridology.* Corona, 2005.

Andrews, John. *Endocrinology & Iridology.* Corona, 2005.

Andrews, John. *Immunology & Iridology.* Corona, 2003.

Colton, James and Sheelagh. *Iridology: Health Analysis and Treatments from the Iris of the Eye.* Shaftesbury, Dorset; Boston, MA: Element, 1996.

Davidson, Victor S. *Iridiagnosis.* HarperCollins Publishers Ltd.,1979.

Deck, Josef. *Differentiation of Iris Diagnosis.* Ettlingen, Germany: Institute for Fundamental Research in Iris Diagnosis, 1983.

Deck, Josef. *Principles of Iris Diagnosis.* Ettlingen, Germany: Institute for Fundamental Research in Iris Diagnosis, 1985.

Jenks, Jim, H.M.D. *The Eyes Have It.* Salt Lake City, UT. Woodland Publishing, Inc., 1995.

Jensen, Bernard, D.C., Ph.D. *The Science and Practice of Iridology, Vol. I.* New Canaan, CT.: Dorothy Hall, Keats Publishing, Inc., 1981.

Lindlahr, Henry, M.D. *Iridiagnosis and Other Diagnostic Methods.* Pomeroy, WA.: Health Research Books, 1974.

Miller, Jonathan D. *Herbs, Iridology and Holistic Health Workbook,* 1982.

Pesek, David J., Ph.D. *Holistic Iridology,* International Institute of Iridology, VHS.

Schmidt, Heinz W. *Iriscopie.* Saarbrucken, Germany, 1989.

Willy Hauser, Josef Karl, and Rudolf Stolz. *Information from Structure and Color.* Felke, 2000.

I suggest that those interested in this fascinating field broaden their knowledge of natural healing. I would like to recommend the following books:

Bar-Sela, Pnina. *Renewal.* Israel: Shachar Ltd., 1998.

Ben-Ari, Yitshak. *Man's Nutrition and His Health.* Self-published, 1994.

Bradshaw, June, *Back to Childhood.*

Jensen, Bernard. *The Science and Practice of Iridology.* Escondido, CA: 1974.

Kloss, Jethro. *Back to Eden* (English). USA: Woodbridge Press, original edition, 1939.

Kushi, Michio. *The Book of Macrobiotics—The Universal Way of Health and Happiness.* Garden City Park, NY: Square One Publishers, 1997.

Manor, Yehuda. *The People of Israel are Alive and Ill.* Self-published, 1993.

Mehlmauer, Leonard, N.D. *The Great Liquid Diet.* Las Vegas, NV: Grand Medicine Press, 2006.

Yakobovich, Avi. *The Green Miracle—Tidings of Health for Humanity.* 2 volumes. Seld Publishing, 2002.

Index

Bold page numbers refer to illustrations and/or photographs.

About the Author

Miriam Garber, Ph.D., is an iridology expert and multidisciplinary therapist with twenty years' experience. She began studying iridology, sclerology, reflexology, and Bach Flower Remedies under the instruction of Dr. Shlomo Schlezinger in 1991. She chose iridology as the "flagship" of her work and broadened her knowledge and study under the instruction of the finest professionals in the international community of iridologists. She also studied sclerology with Dr. Leonard Mehlmauer in the United States and further broadened her knowledge in Ireland, under John Andrews, an international iridology researcher. She was also a student of Zen Buddhism and meditation under the guidance of her mentor, Nissim Amon, and Gudo Wafu Nishijima, a well-known monk and teacher in Japan.

Dr. Garber is a multidisciplinary practitioner in the following fields: reconnective healing, reflexology, IPEC, rebirthing, Reiki, bio-orgonomy, Bach remedies, hands-on therapies, personal awareness, and macrobiotic nutrition.

Israel's leading iridology and sclerology teacher, Dr. Garber dedicates time to research and has achieved several innovative insights. She established a center of natural healing at Moshav Mishmar Hashiva in Israel, which is dedicated to healing people of all ages using natural, noninvasive methods.

Dr. Garber spends most of her time promoting natural healing and invests her experience and energy in treating clients and teaching doctors and other practitioners. She is married and has three children and six grandchildren. She has lived on Moshav Mishmar Hashiva for the past fifty years.

www.ingramcontent.com/pod-product-compliance
Lightning Source LLC
Jackson TN
JSHW071340130125
77033JS00027B/1003